D1250408

THE ULTIMATE PUBLISHING HOUSE (TUPH) US HEADQUARTERS
The Ultimate Publishing House (TUPH)
P.O. Box 1204, Cypress, Texas, U.S.A. 77410

49540 – 80 Glen Shields Avenue, Toronto, Ontario, Canada, L4K 2B0

Telephone: 647-883-1758   Fax: 416-228-2598

www.ultimatepublishinghouse.com and www.adrenalogic.com
E-mail: info@ultimatepublishinghouse.com

US OFFICE: Ordering Information
Quantity Sales: COMPANIES, ORGANIZATIONS, INSTITUTIONS, AND INDUSTRY PUBLICATIONS.

Quantity discounts are available on bulk purchases of this book for reselling, educational purposes, subscription incentives, gifts, sponsorship, or fundraising. Unique books or book excerpts can also be fashioned to suit specific needs such as private labelling with your logo on the cover and a message from or a message printed on the second page of the book. For more information please contact our Special Sales Department at The Ultimate Publishing House.

Orders for college textbook or course adoption use.

Please contact the Ultimate Publishing House
Tel: 647-883-1758
TUPH is a registered trademark of The Ultimate Publishing House

Printed in United States.

Adrenalogic, Outsmarting Stress, by Lena D. Edwards, MD, FAARM

LENA D. EDWARDS, MD, FAARM

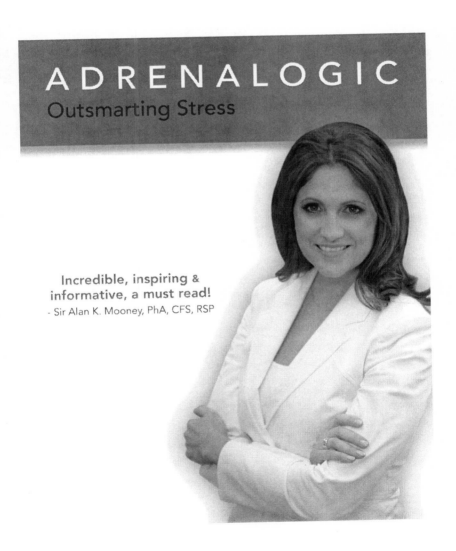

ADRENALOGIC
Outsmarting Stress

Incredible, inspiring &
informative, a must read!
- Sir Alan K. Mooney, PhA, CFS, RSP

DISCLAIMER

Adrenalogic is not intended to diagnose or prescribe any treatment for any medical or psychological condition(s), nor are there any claims or offers to prevent, diagnose, treat, mitigate, or cure any medical or psychological conditions.

The book contains the ideas and opinions of its author and is intended solely to provide helpful information.

It is offered with the understanding that the author and publisher are not engaged in rendering medical, health or any other kind of personal professional services in the book.

The reader should consult his or her medical, health or other competent professional before adopting any of the suggestions in the book.

The author and publisher specifically disclaim all responsibility for any liability, loss, or risk, personal or otherwise, that is incurred as a consequence (directly or indirectly) of the use and application of any of the contents of this book. The book contains the following disclaimer:

The names of people mentioned in the case studies published within the book have been changed to protect the people's identity.

TESTIMONIALS

Incredible, inspiring & informative; a must read!

Sir Alan K. Mooney, PhA, CFS, RSP

"This is a really complex subject even for physicians. Lena has great insight into adrenal health and overall wellness. I certainly understand the concepts better now that I did in medical school. I've recommended it to other physicians and patients."

Michael Banks, MD
Vice President, Co-Founder - THE DOCTOR'S CHANNEL

"A work of art - eloquently written, yet hard hitting at the epicenter of endocrinologic understanding, Adrenalogic is a masterpiece! Dr. Lena (as her patients call her) has brilliantly combined a powerfully profound practical guide for the physician and patient alike. Thorough in her documentation, prolific in academic pursuit and demonstrating a clear concern for our stress-full and hectic 24/7 life-styles, Dr. Edwards has delivered pure genius in Adrenalogic. Certainly transforming right down to and beyond the cellular level, she brings a message of hope for us all."

Dr. Norman D.E. Raymond, D.O., FACOOG,CCD
Obstetrics & Gynecology, Clinical Professor,
Ohio University College of Medicine

"My grandma taught me that the 'proof was in the pudding.' What Dr. Edwards says WORKS! I am now looking forward to my 'back 40' with the same excitement I felt in the first 40 years. Thank you Dr. Edwards! It is all because of you. Length of life is meaningless if it is not quality. I am excited about having a long 'QUALITY' life."

Linda Toupin
National Sales Director - Mary Kay Inc.

"Dr. Edwards has written the most important contemporary work available today on the physiologic and medical aspects of the stress response. No one has assembled such detailed and practical information on the topic in one book. A must read for anyone dealing with stress… which is probably everyone!"

Andrew Heyman, MD, MHSA
Department of Family Medicine - University of Michigan

"Optimum health (synonymous with best possible immune functions, recovery from disease, top fitness, maximum sexual capacity, least rate of cognitive decline and aging) is defined as a state of homeostasis, arrived at by correctly applying some 40 to 50 variables, which can also be grouped together as good health practices. Stress management, as so magnificently discussed by Dr. Edwards in ADRENALOGIC, is one of those good health practices. Proof comes from Telomere research; Telomeres, repeating sub-units at the end of chromosomes are true indicators of longevity and remaining life potential; distress shortens them, and the modalities utilized so logically in Dr. Edward's book lengthen them."

Dr. Hans J. Kugler, PhD
President - International Academy of Anti-Aging Medicine
www.antiagingforme.com
HK Stem Cell Research

"Adrenalogic is a work of synergism and serendipity, of sense and sensitivity. Dr. Edward's remarkable book in the field of adrenal dysfunction takes an evidence-based approach that dispels ante-nodal notions of adrenal fatigue of a by-gone era. The timing couldn't be more perfect as her thorough research and insightful observations logically and scientifically links the adrenal system, as never before, with the many manifestations of chronic disease found in a stressful world. This foundational work is required reading for all who yearn to live a full life of optimized health and wellness today and in the future."

Roger Garcia, D.O., J.D.
Author, Aged to Perfection

TABLE OF CONTENTS

INTRODUCTION

"Reality is the leading cause of stress amongst those in touch with it."

Lily Tomlin (American Actress and Comedian)

Stress... the term has become a predictable part of our daily vocabulary. It's credited for causing everything from divorce to diet disasters. We have come to expect stress as a normal part of our lives, yet we still do not truly understand its complexity nor have we been equipped to deal with its consequences. In fact, the World Health Organization declares that by the year 2020, stress-related bodily disorders will be among the major causes of disability worldwide.

Gaining a better understanding of stress sometimes requires you to take a deep breath and examine what stress may be doing to you. As an internist who's also Board-Certified and Fellowship-Trained in Functional and Regenerative Medicine, I have spent considerable time researching, writing, and speaking on the subject of stress – how it works, what it does to our minds and bodies, and how it affects our lives, our work and our relationships. And, that's not just hyperbole: As a hard-working solo physician and faculty member, small business owner, working mother, and caffeine-devotee, I too have suffered from the mayhem that many of you are experiencing.

Modern-day men and women are stressed, depressed, and distressed. Millions suffer from anxiety, allergies, irritable bowel syndrome, chronic fatigue syndrome, obesity and depression, but a useful diagnosis eludes many of us. I recognize that patients are frequently prescribed expensive pharmaceuticals or self-medicate by taking over-the-counter remedies for their symptoms. And, it's my desire to eradicate this phenomenon by sharing my knowledge about the origins and implications of stress in **Adrenalogic**. Today's quick fix methods may help in the short-term but are unlikely to provide long-term results. It's frustrating and costly for patients, employers and doctors alike.

In 2002, I had an epiphany while sitting in the office of my private practice, elbows deep in patient charts: At the time, I was practicing medicine in a way that was not always improving the lives or longevity of my patients. Instead of being a healer, I felt like a human Band-Aid. As a result, I spent the next several years exploring the fields of integrative, regenerative, and functional medicine. Through my additional training, I developed a better understanding of *why* symptoms and disease states evolve and what proactive steps can be taken to prevent disease. Adding the *why* to the *how* and *what* allowed me not only to enhance patient outcomes but also to encourage patients to take a more proactive stance in their own healthcare.

And so I began to chart a new course for my life and career. I immersed myself in the medical literature published on the topics of stress, health, and disease. I was amazed to discover the sheer volume of material available! It was through this extensive research, my clinical experience, and my interactions with tens of thousands of patients that the vital information included in this book was compiled.

The current facts on stress and its effects on our health should serve as our ultimate wake-up call: We are truly in charge of our own destinies. It is my hope that this book will provide you with timely and accurate information on how stress is affecting you mentally and physically and what steps you can take to outsmart your stress. Furthermore, the information contained in **Adrenalogic** is intended to provide you with a better understanding of how stress can fuel illness and disease development outside the basic concept of "adrenal fatigue" – which is, at best, a misnomer. This book will serve as your evidence-based guide and will provide you with the accurate information and insight you need to take the appropriate steps regaining your health and avoiding disease.

Adrenalogic is written for all of you who may suffer from inexplicable symptoms, such as fatigue, chronic pain, and stress sensitivity, in the face of "normal" test results. You know there is something more going on, but

LENA D. EDWARDS MD, FAARM

you need guidance on where to begin. **Adrenalogic** is your starting point, providing you with the tools you need to empower you to take control of your stress and your health. So, now that you have found a reliable guide to assist you in your journey to better health and vitality, let's begin by taking a better look at the topic of chronic stress and stress induced disease and discuss ways in which you can guide yourself out of the stress maze you may currently find yourself in.

ABOUT THE AUTHOR
DR. LENA D. EDWARDS

Buoyed by numerous awards and more than a decade of training in the fields of internal medicine, hormone restoration therapy, and anti-aging medicine, Dr. Lena Edwards firmly believes in optimizing health and preventing illness by promoting patient awareness. Dr. Edwards' goal in writing Adrenalogic is to empower individuals to better understand the connection between chronic stress and disease and to be proactive in their healthcare.

Honoured as "Intern of the Year" during her residency training at the University of Kentucky School Of Medicine (UKMC) in 1997, Dr. Edwards also served as Chief Resident at UKMC's Department of Internal Medicine. In addition to being trained as an internist, she is both Board Certified and Fellowship Trained in Anti-Aging and Regenerative Medicine and Fellowship Trained in Integrative Cancer Therapy. Less than 2,000 physicians worldwide have this degree of training in the area of Anti-Aging and Regenerative Medicine. In addition to her medical accolades, she was voted "Small Business Women of the Year" in 2008 by the local chapter of the National Association of Women Business Owners.

Using adrenal health as a spring board, Adrenalogic: Outsmarting Stress reveals the link between stress levels and our fundamental health, highlighting the important role the adrenal glands play as part of a larger, more complex system. Written with humor and ample patient case studies, Dr. Edwards applies her abundant experience in this field to enlighten and inform.

Dr. Edwards currently resides with her family in Lexington, Kentucky where she operates her medical practice, Balance Health & Wellness Center. She also serves as a community faculty member for the University of Kentucky Medical Center and is a faculty member for several other prominent medical associations. Dr. Edwards has co-authored numerous published peer-reviewed articles on topics within the realm of anti-aging and functional medicine and, as a member of several national speakers' bureaus, actively delivers presentations to physicians, healthcare professionals and patients around the world.

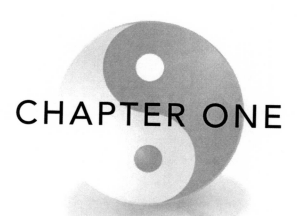

CHAPTER ONE

Red Alert: The Complex Nature Of Stress

According to the World Health Organization, by the year 2020, mental disease, including stress-related disorders will be the second leading cause of disability worldwide.

Does this scenario sound familiar? You're feeling stressed and unwell and decide to see your trusted doctor. After several disappointing visits, rounds of medications, and several weeks, you're still not feeling like yourself. Not fond of using prescription drugs to mask symptoms, you decide to take matters into your own hands and research probable causes. Your research yields some reasonable explanations for your symptoms, and the term "adrenal fatigue" continues to appear, along with suggestions for helpful supplements. Your curiosity presses you, and you start reading about adrenal fatigue. For the first time you think, "A-ha! I knew I wasn't crazy. Finally there's a diagnosis out there that matches my symptoms!" While these particular results lack some important facts, conducting research about symptoms and causes of stress is worthwhile. It is true that your adrenal glands are indeed a part of a very complex stress response system. However, as you continue to read this book, you will come to realize how complex the stress response system is, how stress affects our health and how confining and even inaccurate the term "adrenal fatigue" actually is. It's vitally important to me that I dispel myths and provide you with concrete explanations and reliable solutions. With the proper tools in hand, you will be better equipped to understand your body and take control of your health. You will also be able to use the information in Adrenalogic to work collaboratively with your health care provider to feel your best, prevent disease, and maybe even live longer.

There is much to know about the "great equalizer" we know as stress. When managed wisely, it can provide the motivation and push we need to excel. When poorly managed, it can be our greatest foe. With that in mind, let's take a step back to gain a clear understanding of the evolution of the concept of stress.

THE EVOLUTION OF STRESS

Our species is constantly changing and evolving thanks to daily advancements in the natural world, in science, and in industry. However, we owe much of our current understanding of the concept of stress to the pioneers and forefathers in medicine, education, technology and science. For instance, today, if you were to spurt out advice to a friend using the phrase "mind-body connection," your friend probably wouldn't give it a second thought. But, if you tried saying that a hundred years ago, the same phrase may have caused serious confusion among your friends, perhaps even causing them to be concerned about your sanity.

Today's scientists and medical professionals have a greater understanding and appreciation for stress and the stress response system with which our bodies have been equipped to promote our survival. Integral to our stress response system are the adrenal glands – two small, bean-shaped organs that sit atop the kidneys. The discovery of the adrenal glands and their importance in human health and disease was first described by Thomas Addison in 1855 (hence the term Addison's Disease). Dr. Charles Sajous continued to pursue research within this arena and was the first to coin the term hypoadrenia in the early 1900's. He described hypoadrenia as a state of adrenal gland "exhaustion" in which symptoms of fatigue and susceptibility to infection would arise as a consequence of prolonged strain or labor. He further subdivided hypoadrenia into three stages dependent upon the degree of adrenal gland dysfunction:

- **Functional hypoadrenia** - The adrenals are unable to function properly because of such things as delayed development, old age, or starvation
- **Progressive hypoadrenia** - Internal assaults, such as infections and cancer, progressively shuts down adrenal gland function
- **Terminal hypoadrenia** - "Exhaustion" of the adrenals occurring as a late complication of the initial assault (i.e. infections, cancers, etc.)

It's important to understand that in Sajous's time, the critical contributions of the brain, immune system, and other influential factors in the stress response had not yet been fully appreciated.

Dr. Walter Bradford Cannon, an American psychologist, was also profoundly influential in contributing to the science of stress in the 1920's and 30's. Cannon was the first to describe the concept of the "fight or flight" response, the body's reaction when faced with an immediate threat. He further developed the widely-used term *homeostasis* – internal mechanisms allowing an organism to adjust to external challenges in order to maintain balance. Dr. Cannon is also credited for recognizing that stressors can be both emotional and physical in nature.

The most prominent pioneer of stress research is undeniably "The father of stress," Dr. Hans Selye. While not a moniker that most would wish to possess, Selye's extensive research on physical stressors generated a massive impact on our understanding and appreciation of the stress response. Born in Austria and educated in Rome, Prague and Paris, Selye ended up in Montreal, Quebec, Canada where he joined the endocrinology research team at McGill University. A diligent researcher, Selye shed light on the extreme effect of stress on our bodies.

"Stress is the nonspecific response of the body to any demand. A stressor is an agent that produces stress at any time. The general adaptation syndrome (GAS) represents the chronologic development of the response to stressors when their activation is prolonged. It consists of three phases: the alarm reaction, the stage

of resistance, and the state of exhaustion."

Hans Selye, "Forty Years of Stress Research," 1976

As Hans Selye proclaims in his article, *Forty Years of Stress Research: Principal Remaining Problems and Misconceptions*, "Stress is the salt of life; few people would like to live an existence of no runs, no hits, no errors. Yet it is beneficial for the human machine to rest periodically; hence the development of various religious and psychologic techniques designed to diminish temporarily all forms of biologic stress, close to the minimum compatible with survival. Total elimination of stress - that is, cessation of demands made upon any part of the body, including the cardiovascular, respiratory and nervous systems - would be equivalent to death."

These vitally important historical contributions over the past century and a half have allowed today's clinicians to better understand how stress causes everything from PMS to premature aging.

The General Adaptation Syndrome was a milestone theory postulated by Selye. The graph above illustrates the basic tenets of this concept. Disturbance of balance (or homeostasis) initially causes an alarm reaction which, left unchecked can lead to resistance (or 'adaptation'). However, over time, an organism will eventually succumb to exhaustion under the influence of chronic stress. The optimum opportunity for intervention for humans dealing with stress is smack between "alarm" and "exhaustion" – at the tipping point of chronic stress if you will.

Since Selye, there have been many profoundly influential clinicians and researchers who have contributed to our understanding of stress-induced disease. However, there is one individual in particular I want to make special mention of, modern-day researcher Bruce McEwen. Dr. McEwen, a professor of Neuroscience at Rockefeller University, expounds on the concepts of stress by defining the terms *allostasis* and *allostatic load*. His definitions explain how various types of long-term stress cause wear and tear (allostatic load) on our systems which may result in a new but sometimes dysfunctional balance (allostasis) under the influence of this allostatic load. His work suggests that stressful situations are distinctive in that each person adjusts or habituates to repeated stress differently.

So, while one person's nightmare may include speaking at a public conference in front of three hundred people, another person may have done it so frequently that she barely bats an eyelash upon stepping on to the stage.

Dr. McEwen reminds modern-day healthcare providers about patient stress and the potential complications thereof by suggesting that, "Physicians and other healthcare providers can help patients reduce allostatic load by helping them learn coping skills, recognize their own limitations, and relax." Sane and simple solutions to a larger-than-life problem which aligns with the wise words of Dr. William Osler: "It is much more important to know what sort of patient has a disease than what sort of disease a patient has."

BE YOUR OWN HEALTHCARE ADVOCATE

Western medicine is making huge strides in understanding and appreciating the ancillary benefits of integrative medicine modalities such as naturopathy, chiropractic, acupuncture, Chinese medicine, massage therapy, and homeopathy. However, if you're counting on your doctor to make these connections for you, you may be out of luck. In addition to time constraints often overshadowing medical appointments, there is a definite "disconnect" between traditional and integrative medicine approaches when it comes to stress-induced medical conditions.

In addition, doctors don't traditionally receive a great deal of training on the topic of stress during medical school, even though we could all pose as poster children on the topic! I know that I received very little instruction during my traditional medical training on stress, the stress response system, and how chronically abnormal levels of stress hormones adversely affect patients. Only after spending the past five years researching, writing, and speaking on this topic have I fully realized this void and, truthfully, I'm amazed that my medical training was so deficient in this area.

Clearly, I'm not the only one who thinks this way. As George A. Perdrizet writes in his article, *Hans Selye: Responses to Stress*: "*Despite the wide-reaching implications of the stress response as recognized by Dr. Selye,*

I am puzzled by the lack of emphasis given to his work by educators in modern medical and bio-medical sciences."

While troubling, this news should empower and prompt all of us, patients and doctors alike, to be advocates in healthcare delivery and education. Medicine evolves constantly. As such, doctors, while compassionate and well-educated, are not necessarily all-knowing. In *Adrenalogic*, I hope to give you a better understanding of how your body works and how all hormones, including stress hormones, work in conjunction with each other under the profound influence of your lifestyle, habits, behavior, work environment, exercise patterns, and diet to affect how you feel and how you age.

The great news is that medicine truly is changing, and the realization that Western medicine is not the penultimate for all treatment continues to emerge. Over seventy medical school programs in this country now have integrative medicine programs including Duke, the University of Michigan, MD Anderson Cancer Center, and the Mayo Clinic, just to name a few. As ancient medical philosophies are revisited and new medical practices emerge, patients can expect to see healthcare professionals that are more knowledgeable and open to exploring non-conventional medical approaches to patient care. It is within this new context that the importance of stress and stress-related disease, aging, and premature death is being fully realized. And although I am furthering this goal by continuing to write, teach, and speak on this topic, there is definitely power in numbers.

Finally, before Chapter One comes to a close, I want to show you how complicated our stress response systems can be by using a patient case study to illustrate my point— and you'll find a myriad of patient case studies in *Adrenalogic*. This has been done to provide readers with a robust picture of stress and health. Perhaps you'll see yourself or a family member in one of the case studies.

This particular case focuses on "Judy," a nineteen-year-old female college freshman who had become so ill that she could no longer function at college. After seeing several physicians who prescribed common medications and speculated on plausible diagnoses, an unwell and frustrated Judy and her mother finally came to see me.

JUDY'S STORY

"I went to see Dr. Edwards because my mother heard about her through a friend. I guess I decided to see her because nothing that my regular doctors were doing was making me feel any better. I didn't have any health problems or take any medications at the time I went to see Dr. Edwards. My other doctors had tried to put me on sleeping pills and anti-depressant medications, but my mother would not hear of it.

I felt fine until about four months before going to see Dr. Edwards. I had graduated from high school and was working a summer job as a life guard before college. I started my freshman year at a college about one hour away from home. I was nervous because I had never lived away from home, and I was going to have to share a dorm room with two other girls that I didn't know. I had a very hard time keeping up with a full schedule, and I couldn't sleep at night thinking about the tests I would have to take the next day. I skipped meals all the time either because I was too busy to eat or because I did not like the food.

A few months after starting school, I got my first cold. It took me about two weeks to get over it. One month later, I got sick again. Except this time, I was really sick. I was coughing, achy, and feverish. I was exhausted during the day, I could not sleep at night, I continued to lose weight, and my whole body hurt. I went to Student Health and they gave me an antibiotic which didn't help. Then, my mother came and took me to my regular doctor. That doctor just gave me more antibiotics and some other medicines for my symptoms. But even after taking all of it, I still did not feel better.

Then, my mother took me to her doctor. He did some blood work and a chest x-ray and told me that "everything was fine." He said I probably had a virus and that my symptoms would eventually go away. The cough and fever did, but everything else stuck around. I could not take any time off because I had already missed so much school. Two more weeks went by and then I went back to Student Health. The physician assistant said

I was depressed and gave me a prescription for an anti-depressant. I tried to tell her that I was not depressed. I had felt fine until I got sick. She said that the "stress of college was just getting to me" and that the medication would help with that. When I called my mother later that day to tell her, she told me not to take the anti-depressants. She said she had found out about Dr. Edwards and was coming to get me from college and take me to her office. At that point, I felt so bad that I agreed to go.

By the time I saw Dr. Edwards, I felt horrible. I had all the same symptoms I had before except now my periods were irregular and my hair had started to fall out. When I first saw Dr. Edwards, she asked me a lot of questions and examined me. She also ordered a lot of blood work and a saliva test. I had never heard of a saliva test before. She said it was a very good way to check my stress hormone levels. She said that blood tests would only show a problem if my adrenal glands were completely "shot." She told me that if my stress hormone levels were abnormal then we would need to figure out possible causes.

After three weeks, we went back to see Dr. Edwards to review my test results. My tests showed that I had a mono infection that was not going away. My thyroid hormone levels were low, my B12 and Vitamin D levels were very low, and I was slightly anemic. My saliva test showed that I was not making enough cortisol during the day to give me energy. Dr. Edwards explained that it was hard to tell what caused the problem because there were so many things wrong on my labs. She explained how anything that stressed my body could cause cortisol levels to be abnormal, and that once the stress hormones were low, everything would be worse. She suspected the mono infection may have been the cause of the low cortisol levels during the day. She also told me that my cortisol levels at night were probably higher than normal and that was why I was having trouble sleeping. Basically, my levels were "backwards," and needed to get back to normal in order for me to feel better.

Dr. Edwards started me on a good quality multi-vitamin since I was not eating very well. I also got extra Vitamin D, B-12 shots, and iron to cover the low levels. She also gave me Phosphatidylserine [see Chapter Nine for more information] to take at bedtime to help me to stay asleep and a supplement with plant adaptogens to take during the day to help with focus and energy. I got some L-Theanine [see Chapter Nine for more information] to help with my anxiety and focus which worked great and did not make me sleepy at all. I also received a prescription for an anti-viral medication for my Epstein Barr virus infection and some thyroid medication for low thyroid. She also recommended I take the semester off so I could focus on getting better. She helped me with my diet and told me to focus more on combining protein with complex carbohydrates and eating small, frequent meals to keep my cortisol levels steady.

Within three weeks, I was beginning to feel better. Dr. Edwards saw me once a month and continued to do follow-up tests. She discovered some other vitamin deficiencies and adjusted my supplements. She never gave me a prescription for an anti-depressant or a sleeping pill. After three months, I started having normal periods again. My hair stopped falling out and I was actually sleeping through the night. I started gaining some weight back and my energy levels improved. Dr. Edwards explained that finding the cause of the symptoms was the real key to getting me better but that all of the other problems that had cropped up during that time also needed to be fixed.

At first, she advised that I go back to school part-time. I did fine during that period so after a few weeks, I was back to full-time. At that point, I was only taking a multi-vitamin because I did not need the other supplements and vitamins any more. When she re-tested all of my hormone levels, they were much better. My repeat saliva testing showed my cortisol patterns were back to near normal levels. Dr. Edwards made me promise not to overdo it so I would not get sick again. That was kind of hard to do because it was so nice to finally feel better! So now, I am a semester behind in school. But at least I was able to go back. Without Dr. Edwards' help, I don't think I could have finished college."

Considering all we've covered in Chapter One, are you more aware of the complex nature of the stress response system, and its all-encompassing influence over our health? I hope that the data and shared knowledge has sparked some new connections for you. Let's move on to Chapter Two where we discuss stress in more detail – how it helps and how it hurts.

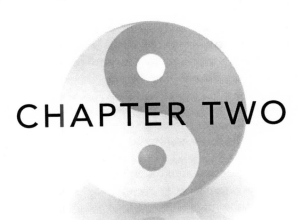

CHAPTER TWO

Fight Or Flight: How Our Stress Response System Originated

"Man should not try to avoid stress any more than he would shun food, love or exercise."

Hans Selye

Relatively speaking, we've only just begun to explore and truly appreciate the prevailing force we know as stress. It's a subject so vital and compelling that I could easily devote thousands of pages to its analysis. However, in the interest of time, I've dedicated this chapter to delving into some of the most pressing issues surrounding stress by providing a deeper understanding of the fight or flight phenomenon and how it can go awry, the positive attributes of stress, and the trickle-down effect of chronic stress on our bodies.

OUR EARLIEST ANCESTORS EXPERIENCED IT, TOO

In Chapter One, we explained how, a century ago, Dr. Walter Cannon identified the term "fight or flight," a description which is still apt today.

Now, originally, the term "stress" was meant to describe anything causing a disruption in internal balance. Since for every action there is an equal and opposite reaction, disruption of balance leads to an instinctive need to re-balance. The re-balancing act involves either defending your position (fight) or changing your surroundings (flight).

Historically, this response has proven essential as humans (and other animals) were obliged to deal with impending doom at a moments notice. To illustrate, humor me for a moment as we go back in time 10,000 or so years. Now, picture yourself as a caveman (or woman). As you bemoan the lack of a heat source and your rough-hewn rock tools, picture a large, snarling animal eyeing your food. Imminent danger! Within a nanosecond, your brain perceives the stress and signals your adrenal glands to produce epinephrine, norepinephrine, and cortisol.

These hormones then work their way through your body, making your heart beat faster, your blood pressure rise, your body stand more erect, and your jaw and fists clench. Back then, instinct only allowed two choices... fight or flight. Times and intellect have clearly affected the way we now think, perceive, and behave, and this has only complicated our otherwise rudimentary stress response. Cave people didn't need to worry about who was going to pick the children up from school or if their boss was going to fire them before the holidays.

Unlike our cave dwelling counterparts, we have far more sophisticated worries – we must now decide whether to stand our ground and physically (or verbally) hash it out or whether to use that same burst of anxious energy to high-tail it out of a physically or mentally dangerous situation. We endure stress in our jobs, in our relationships, and in our environments that were not in existence thousands of years ago.

But, regardless of the stress, the physical response has always remained the same. That initial burst or shock of stress, the "adrenaline rush" is the same hormonal reaction that occurs when your boss comes barging into your office unhappy with a report you just turned in or when you nearly crash into the car in front of you because you are too busy talking on your cell phone.

LENA D. EDWARDS MD, FAARM

By design, our body has the ability to protect itself from short-term stress with the built-in conditioning of our fight or flight response. That gives us, say, thirty minutes or so to deal with a stressful situation. Unfortunately, the torment of many of our modern stressors is not short and sweet but rather long, painful, and repetitive. And although our bodies do a phenomenal job at keeping us alive under the influence of chronic stress, we are much worse for the wear. We will elaborate on this further towards the end of this chapter.

MY STRESS IS NOT YOUR STRESS

One of the things that makes humans unique is the fact that we all feel and exhibit emotions differently even in the same situation. For example, you and a friend meet up for dinner and to see the latest horror movie. Your friend has an extreme reaction to the film — screaming with terror throughout while you yawn and look around the theater, not sure what all the fuss is about. Why would he react this way when you don't find the horror scenes compelling?

The same thing occurs with many other types of stress — one woman's stressful situation is another woman's exciting challenge. Why the difference? There are a variety of factors to consider; some of the main ones are:

- **Childhood development** — Separation from parents and parental neglect also cause major stress and developmental damage to babies and children as secure parental bonds are of utmost importance to healthy development.
- **Body size at birth** — Low birth weight means that a child is already at a disadvantage in his ability to fight off infection and "catch up" to his peers.
- **Perinatal malnutrition** — If a woman smokes, takes drugs or alcohol or consumes a poor diet while pregnant, this can cause a variety of mental and physical problems in the fetus.
- **In-utero environment** — While a child is in utero (in her mother's womb), a calm, stress and toxin-free environment is key to healthy development.
- **Abuse** — Abuse of any kind — mental, physical, verbal, sexual, can

seriously impact a person's stress level and damage the normal workings of the fight or flight response.

- **Isolation** – Humans are meant to interact with each other. Isolation for prolonged periods of time results in increased stress in many.

According to a 2007 study in *American Academy of Child and Adolescent Psychiatry*, "In humans, the most well-documented consequences of prenatal stress are preterm birth and low birth weight. Accumulating evidence suggests that the effects of prenatal maternal stress persist into the postpartum period and that consideration of the timing of exposures will be essential to our understanding of the influence of prenatal stress."

If you're wondering about why you react the way you do, the influence of these factors should shed some light. In fact, a substantial amount of research has shown how impactful these early life experiences are in not only shaping who you are as an individual but also in solidifying your stress response system for life.

Other factors that influence activity of our stress response systems include:

- **Age:** Older age brings about gradual deterioration of all organs and systems, including those involved in the stress response. Consequently, HPA axis dysfunction is more common as we age.
- **Gender:** Studies have shown that women have more HPA axis dysfunction than do men. Although the reasons are not fully understood, Dr. Bruce McEwen, whom we introduced earlier, states: "The decline in estrogen secretion at menopause increases the activity of the HPA axis, a development that has been linked to greater cognitive decline among elderly women than among elderly men."

THE BENEFITS OF STRESS

Stop! Before you "stress out" about stress, please realize that it's not all bad news. The complete absence of stress is not healthy either. A certain level of stress is essential in allowing us to reach our full physical and mental potential. As shown in the graph below, "good stress" (eustress)

LENA D. EDWARDS MD, FAARM

in the short term can actually improve our performance and productivity. I'll remind you of the quote from Hans Selye, "Stress is the salt of life; few people would like to live an existence of no runs, no hits, no errors…"

THE HUMAN FUNCTION CURVE

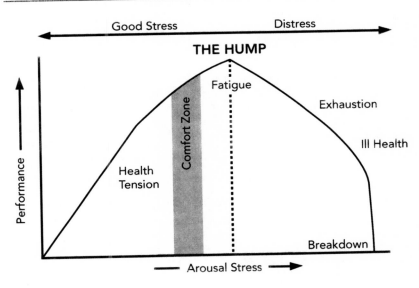

Adapted from: Nixon, P: Practioner, 1979

Distress is the word we typically use to describe negative types of stress – divorce, loss of a loved one, or financial constraints. Conversely, "eustress," a term coined by Hans Selye in 1975, is the optimal form of stress, usually related to desirable events in a person's life.

Eustress gives us meaning and purpose. It keeps us goal-oriented and focused on a greater good. Getting a bonus for a job well done or winning an award qualify as types of eustress. The effects of both eustress and distress are cumulative and can be equally taxing on the body. The end result ultimately depends upon on a person's perception and way of adapting to the change that has caused the stress. The body itself cannot physically tell the difference between distress and eustress. As such, numerous other influences such as our upbringing, our beliefs, our perceptions, and our personalities are vital in determining the outcome.

The type of stress and a person's perception to it greatly influences the body's reaction to the stressful event. Take, for example, the 2008 U.K. study of nurses published in the *Journal of Advanced Nursing* which found that nursing students who coped well (describing their experiences as "eustressful" instead of distressful) drew on effective support networks and adopted a positive, optimistic perspective towards program issues.

THE DAMAGING SIDE OF STRESS

So, we now know that stress is multifaceted and can even be beneficial if managed correctly. However, the negative aspects of stress are, unfortunately, so rampant and insidious that they can crop up daily for many people around the world – making the need for knowledge that much more important.

In my opinion, family gatherings tend to be the perfect environment to analyze stress at its best. To better illustrate a typical stress response situation, think about the latest family gathering you took part in. Was it smooth sailing or were there rocky waters to contend with? Does the following scenario sound at all familiar?

There you are, wearing your expensive new outfit at the Thanksgiving Day table with a dozen other family members. The day starts off well but, across the table, you find your mother-in-law staring you down, ready to continue an argument started many months ago. Your catecholamines and cortisol (among other hormones) are up. As your mother-in-law's eyes burn you with a fiery stare, you feel your chest get tight and your underarms dampen.

Rather than letting the words fly in front of a myriad family members, you jump up and go for a walk (a flight response). It feels good to get some fresh air plus, you now know that exercise is a eustress. After returning from the walk, you feel better and are ready to move on. However, while you were gone, your mother-in-law chose to sit and stew (distress).

So what is going on with your stress response system in the thirty minutes in which your argument resumes? Your adrenals have received the memo and are cranking out cortisol so that your body has everything it needs in the form of fuel, focus, and endurance to flee… but what about three hours or three days later?

Let's review cortisol's functions:

- It diverts the body's essential resources into promoting survival
- It causes blood sugar, pulse, and blood pressure to rise
- It dampens immune defenses
- It shuts down reproductive functions
- It causes a reduction in stomach acid production and an increase in elimination of food in the intestinal tract so your system will not be distracted by digestion
- It heightens your brain awareness, so no sleep for you
- It suppresses growth hormone production (who cares about growth and repair of tissues in the face of death or major stress!)
- It reduces thyroid hormone activity by decreasing production and inactivating circulating thyroid hormone

Clearly, these adaptive responses are beneficial in the short term. But what can we expect when the hormone initially designed to protect us from imminent death eventually becomes the cause in the long run? The research on stress-mediated diseases to date is quite clear—diabetes, high blood pressure, heart disease, stroke, cancers of all types, infertility, obesity, metabolic syndrome, inflammation, mood disorders, osteoporosis, and irritable bowel syndrome are but a few of the diseases you can potentially look forward to developing.

As you begin to examine how your stressors are affecting you on a personal level, let us extend the scope even further and turn to how stress and stress-related diseases affect us on a larger scale.

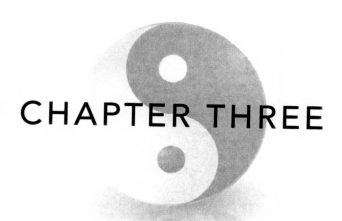

CHAPTER THREE

Turbulence! Understanding Stress And Society

"Oh, you hate your job? Why didn't you say so? There's a support group for that. It's called EVERYBODY, and they meet at the bar."

Drew Carey

Rushing out of the office where you've been working late – again – you collect your bags from the tiny cubicle where you've been sitting all day typing on the computer and breathing recycled air. Stumbling outside, you pass a group of colleagues huddled together smoking cigarettes in front of the building. Waving good-bye to them, you rush down the littered sidewalk, past the music store booming tunes from speakers and into the subway station. You catch the last train which is filled to the brim with frazzled administrative assistants, impatient mothers of small children, and college kids hitting the bars for a night on the town. Pressed up against your fellow stressed out commuters, you patiently wait until your stop is announced then proceed to run like crazy down the street to collect your two kids from daycare; miraculously, you're only one minute late!

The above scenario may not fit *your life* exactly; you may drive a truck or teach high school students or stay home with your children or work out

LENA D. EDWARDS MD, FAARM

of doors. However, if you live and work in the Western world, you'll be subjected to the effects of environmental and societal stress regardless of your daily routine.

According to the *American Institute of Stress*:

- 43 percent of all adults suffer adverse health effects due to stress.
- 75 to 90 percent of all visits to primary care physicians (PCPs) are for stress-related complaints or disorders.
- An estimated one million workers are absent on an average work day due to stress-related complaints. Stress is believed to be responsible for more than half of the 550 million workdays lost annually because of absenteeism.
- Stress has been linked to all the leading causes of death, including heart disease, cancer, lung ailments, cirrhosis of the liver, and suicide.
- Nearly half of all American workers suffer from symptoms of burnout, a disabling consequence of stress on the job.
- Work place violence is rampant. There are almost two million reported instances of homicide, aggravated assault, rape, or sexual assault. Homicide is the second leading cause of fatal occupational injury and the leading cause of death for working women.

We've already defined several terms related to stress. However, let us further delineate the meaning and types of chronic stress:

Chronic continuous stress: Continuous exposure (days or weeks) to stressful situation

Chronic repeated intermittent stress: Repeated daily exposure to the same stressor (for 30 minutes to 4 hours) for one or more weeks

Chronic variable stress: Chronic exposure to variable daily stressors

Perhaps you have come to embrace your various types of chronic stress as a normal part of your life. As someone who's studied this phenomenon in great detail and personally experienced it, I'm here to tell you that, while chronic stress seems to have become an iconic element in our society, it is absolutely not, nor will it ever be, normal.

Although *Adrenalogic* focuses primarily on the **health consequences** of chronic stress, taking a step back to understand how stress affects various external aspects of our lives makes its role that much more compelling. Let me elaborate a bit more on the major causes of societal and environmental stress.

STRESS IN THE WORKPLACE

Have you heard the term "going postal?" It's not at all a light-hearted statement but, if you heard someone say it, you'd know immediately that they were having a very bad day at work. Sadly, it's an accurate portrayal of how many workers feel day after day. It may reassure you to know that you are not alone and to understand that workplace stress affects us all.

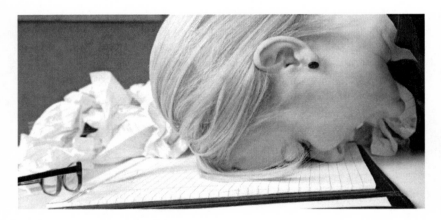

What is workplace stress exactly? *The National Institute of Occupations Safety and Health (NIOSH)* defines it as, "the harmful physical and emotional responses that occur when the requirements of the job do not match the capabilities, resources, or needs of the worker." Simply put, this means that when work overwhelms us, we get incredibly stressed out.

Here are some facts about stress in the workplace:
- In 1992, a United Nations Report labeled job stress "The 20th Century Disease."
- A few years later, the World Health Organization claimed job stress

LENA D. EDWARDS MD. FAARM

to be a "World Wide Epidemic."

- A 2002 *Aventis Healthcare* survey in Canada found 51 percent of employees experienced "much stress" at work, with 25 percent of them succumbing to physical illness as a direct consequence.
- In Japan, the term "karoshi" has been coined to describe sudden death due to job stress. Since the late 1980's, this condition has received so much attention that major Japanese corporations have adjusted work environments accordingly.
- The *Australian Psychological Society* reported that in 2002, stress accounted for over half of all long term (twelve or more weeks) compensation claims among Australian workers that did not involve an injury.

In our "work more, stress more, earn less" society, late nights at the office, burn-out, stress-induced disability leave, disability payouts, and work place rampages have become increasingly common. During your next coffee break, consider some basic statistics cited by *The National Institute of Occupational Safety and Health*:

- 40 percent of workers feel their job is very or extremely stressful
- 25 percent view their jobs as the number one stressor in their lives
- 75 percent of employees believe that workers have more on-the-job stress than a generation ago
- 29 percent of workers feel "quite a bit" or extremely stressed at work
- 26 percent of workers are "often or very often burned out or stressed by their work"
- Job stress is more strongly associated with health complaints than financial or family issues

Why do we let ourselves "go there?" When times are tough, many people are grateful to have a job and bring in a steady income. We do not want to risk getting laid off or fired so we work the extra hours or juggle too many tasks. There's also the basic human characteristic of competition: if Maria got promoted because she works harder and faster, then I better do the same. This can be a good thing if it drives us to excel, but it can it can easily backfire – forcing people away from down time, friends, family and rest.

The specific sources of job stress are many but seem to be directly related to the number of hours worked, dangerous or unpleasant working conditions, poor social environment, and job insecurity.

In addition to the costs on our health and psyche directly caused by job stress, the economy takes an equally huge hit from such indirect costs as:

- Accidents
- Absenteeism
- Employee turnover
- Diminished productivity
- Legal costs

To elaborate, **among American workers, job stress accounts for absenteeism rates of 19 percent and job turnover rates of 40 percent.** The Bureau of Labor statistics estimates the median absence from such stress-induced absence at twenty-three days, **four times the level of all nonfatal occupational injuries and illnesses.** Additionally, 60 percent of worker compensation awards are related to stress.

To supplement these indirect expenditures, the direct medical costs subsequent to job related stress are equally mind-boggling (data from: National Foundation of Brain Research, NIOSH, Harvard Business Review):

- Healthcare expenditures are nearly 50 percent greater for workers who report high levels of stress
- $171 billion dollars spent annually
  - $145 billion for injuries
  - $26 billion for diseases
- 15 American workers die daily from an injury suffered at work
- 134 American workers die daily from work-related diseases
- Depression, a common problem among workers, costs the US $44 billion per year in lost productivity
- 38 American workers develop work-related diseases
- 11,000 American workers are treated in emergency departments for work-related injury and disease daily

In 2002, the journal *Metabolism* noted, **"The disability caused by [job] stress is just as great as the disability caused by workplace accidents or other common medical conditions such as hypertension, diabetes, and arthritis."**

Understanding the enormous weight that job stress puts on individuals, tax payers and families, now is an ideal time to introduce you to Owen.

OWEN'S STORY

Owen was a twenty-six-year-old man who looked like he was going on thirty-eight. He was already showing signs of aging despite the fact the he was supposed to be at the physiological prime of his life. He had graduated from a small town high school and from there moved directly into what he considered to be his lifelong profession: assembly line work at a major automotive manufacturing company.

Owen had come to see me because he was "stressed and tired." He had seen the physician at his place of employment and was told he was "fine." He had tried three different anti-depressants all of which caused side effects and did not improve his depression. Furthermore, he told me he had "no reason to be depressed." He had felt perfectly well until two years ago. He was currently working fifty hours per week, had no financial constraints, had a girlfriend he adored, and had great relationships with his family. He did not drink alcohol but did smoke about a pack of cigarettes daily. He ate a relatively unhealthy diet of fast food because it was convenient, and his work schedule did not allow him much extra time to exercise.

At Owen's initial visit with me, I spent a great deal of time gathering as much history as I could. The patient will always tell you what their diagnosis is (indirectly) if you simply ask enough of the right questions. Owen had always been healthy, no surgeries, no major medical problems, and no chronic medications. He had gone to work at the factory when he was nineteen years old, and his work required him to be exposed to different types of chemicals and loud noises (although he wore the appropriate protective gear). He worked twelve hours shifts, rarely took breaks, and stood for most of the time.

Owen recalls that for the past three years, his work schedule had changed, and he was now working the third shift. His new work hours required him to start work at 5 pm and work until 5 am. Since the days of the week he worked varied, he was never able to maintain a normal schedule. He was already feeling run down at the time his schedule change, but he noticed that many of his symptoms worsened thereafter. He was suffering from insomnia for which he has taking over-the-counter sleep aids. His energy levels during his new "daytime" dwindled and he could not focus. Sex, stamina, and sensibility were all gone.

Owen's initial test results were not surprising. His stressors started much earlier in the form of poor dietary habits, smoking, and his sedentary lifestyle. His stress response system was then further disrupted by his fifty-hour work week and the constant physical demands to which he was exposed. Add to that third shift work, and you end up with Owen's dilemma: the lab results of a person three times his age!

Owen's testosterone and DHEA levels were low, his cortisol levels were backwards (high when they were supposed to be low and vice versa), his melatonin level was low (which can cause sleep disruption and premature aging) as were his growth hormone and thyroid hormone levels. Not surprising, right? Since hormones are released at particular times and in particular patterns, Owen's hormones had no idea when to be released since his sleep wake cycle was constantly changing. His constant state of fight or flight demanded his body to focus its attention upon surviving rather than thriving… Hence, no sex, no energy, no focus, and no sleep. With regards to his memory loss, what Owen also did not realize was that if cortisol levels are elevated over prolonged periods of time, damage occurs to the area of the brain that controls memory, the hippocampus (there is some evidence in the medical research to suggest this change may be irreversible in the face of chronic stress).

The defining moment for Owen's physical and mental demise was his change in schedule to third shift. Significant research has been done on the detrimental effects of third shift work on both health and work performance. Workers who work on a variable shift schedule (and hence disruption of their normal circadian rhythms) experience more physical

LENA D. EDWARDS MD, FAARM

complaints (i.e. headaches, depression, fatigue, lack of concentration), health problems (such as heart disease and cancer), and increased rates of errors and accidents on the job. As such, in addition to prescribing a gradual change in his lifestyle (smoking, eating habits, etc.), I also had to write a letter to Owen's employer restricting Owen from engaging in any third shift work. As long as Owen worked a variable schedule, his internal clock would be perpetually disrupted, he would never feel good, and he would risk future health problems.

Within two months of Owen reverting back to a daytime work schedule of no more than forty hours per week, he was feeling "50 percent better." I prescribed several supplements including melatonin to help his body's internal clock realign itself back to normal. His test results three months later showed improvement in all previous hormone abnormalities, simply from reducing his work related stress! Owen is the perfect example of someone who did not need exotic testing, expensive pharmaceutical drugs, or hormone replacement. His body was already well-equipped to fend for itself and simply needed the correct environment in which to do so.

Help is available to those of you who can relate to Owen's situation. There are excellent resources to help guide you to "busting" job stress and offer advice and assistance. You will find a listing of resources at the end of this book.

SOCIETY'S RESPONSE TO STRESS & BIG PHARMA

How do we solve our problems related to stress? We use drugs. Nearly half of all Americans take at least one prescription drug and over one-third take at least two drugs. In many of these cases, prescription drugs fail to address the true underlying problem, cause adverse side effects, inadequately treat symptoms, and lead to approximately 106,000 deaths annually. Sleep disturbances are one of the most commonly reported symptoms of stress. Nearly half of the U.S. population reports stress-disrupted sleep citing concerns over money and employment as the primary reasons. In fact, sleep aids are used by 16 percent of Americans with difficulty sleeping. Since "symptoms often equals drugs" the pharmaceutical companies thrive in our modern medical predicament. In fact, according to Fortune 500's Industry Rankings, pharmaceutical manufacturing was the most profitable industry in the U.S. from 1995 to 2002, and in 2008 it ranked third with profits after taxes of about 19 percent. From 1999 to 2009, the number of prescriptions purchased in the United States increased 39 percent even though the U.S. population grew only 9 percent. Furthermore, prescription drug sales were $300.3 billion in 2009 and IMS Health forecasts a 3 percent to 6 percent annual growth in the U.S. pharmaceutical market in the next five years, reaching $360 to $390 billion in 2014! Due to the significant overlap in stress-related bodily disorders, it is difficult to accurately quantify the economic burden to society of specific pharmaceutical agents. What is known is that Americans spend approximately $86 billion dollars annually on anti-depressants and around eight billion dollars on medications to treat insomnia. If you were to examine "America's Most Wanted" list of prescription drugs, you would find the pain medication **Vicodin** to be numero uno.

Rounding out the Top 20 are:

- #12 Xanax (anti-anxiety)
- #14 Zoloft (anti-depressant)
- #19 Ambien (insomnia)

(Forbes.com)

Are we stuck in a consumer-driven, quick fix society forever? Will North Americans continue down this road now that we know so much about the terrible burden stress carries and the importance of work/life balance and general happiness? Although this knowledge is not new, some societies have been slow to embrace change. The positive news is that change is in the air as evidenced by the emergence of numerous global non-profit organizations with missions to combat the global stress pandemic. The next section discusses an example of a fresh perspective.

BATTLING STRESS THE NORDIC WAY

To turn the tables, let's focus on a part of the world where levels of both happiness and productivity are high– Scandinavia. The Nordic countries which include Sweden, Denmark, Iceland, Finland, and Norway are known as a hub of innovation, productivity and work/life balance.

Troels Theill Eriksen, Martin Kruse and Gitte Larsen, authors of the business article, *The Scandinavian Way*, summarize this mode of working and living: "When Europe needs vision, it looks increasingly often to the Nordic area. The countries to the north have managed to create a welfare system with free education, public support plans, and a well-developed public health service. The Nordic countries top the international rankings of the most competitive regions in the world despite their having some of the highest taxes in the world, and despite their workers working fewer hours than those of almost any other country. Measured in GNP per capita, the Nordic region, if defined as one country, is among the richest in the world, surpassed only be Luxembourg, Switzerland and Ireland.

How is this possible? Erikson, Kruse and Larsen go on to explain thoroughly. Factors include the use of a democratic management style in most Scandinavian businesses. This means that managers enter into discussions with subordinates to achieve consensus and work to create "productivity, employee happiness, and collegiality among the staff."

In addition, "Scandinavians from childhood are taught to think independently and critically. Nordic employees have developed their professional skills out of personal interest and not from the likelihood of getting a job or good salary. That gives a high level of competence and some of the world's most motivated workers. That combination is particularly important because research into creativity shows that the combination of strong qualifications and motivation is required for creativity and, in the end, innovation."

Need more convincing of Nordic triumph? According to Forbes magazine, Iceland is the world's healthiest country. "Icelanders enjoy one of the world's highest healthy life expectancies. The country is also one of the world's least polluted... and also has one of the highest physician densities, 3.62 per 1,000 people." (Forbes.com, 2008 World's Healthiest Countries).

STRESS IN THE ENVIRONMENT

You might not think much about the belching smoke-stack down the street from your apartment building, the constant racket coming from the screaming sirens racing by your office building, or the bright, unnaturally orange candies you pop in your mouth. Realize that stress does not have to come in the form of a fight with your spouse or a bad day at work. Environmental stressors are equally important in causing disease and premature death.

An environmental stressor is any type of force or event in our environments that causes our bodies to mount a stress response. Given the fact that most disease is acquired from your environment and not your DNA, a discussion about environmental stress is clearly worthwhile. Modern day environmental stressors come in many forms. Here are some of them:

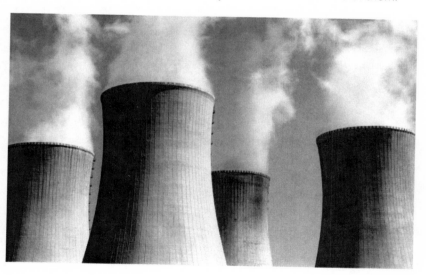

- **Pollution**
  - Air
  - Water
  - Noise
  - Land

- **Radiation**
  - Consumer products
  - Medical (accounts for 50 percent)
  - Radon
  - Cosmic
- **Food and water sources**
  - Additives/preservatives
  - Contamination
  - Highly processed/transformed
- **Medications**
  - Prescription
  - Over the counter
- **Local environment**
  - Classroom over crowding
  - Work place environment
  - Home environment
  - Heavy metal contaminants in air, food, water

Like many things in life, we sometimes get used to (or desensitized to) environmental hazards. Living in an urban setting may mean dealing with crazy traffic and cranky passersby which we sometimes need to "tune out." But, an abundance of stressful factors without time to relax and unwind – away from pollution and noise – causes wear and tear on our mental and physical health.

Over the past several decades, concerted steps have been taken to address and reduce our exposure to environmental stressors. Worldwide, governments have taken measures to limit emissions of carbon dioxide and other greenhouse gases in order to reduce air pollution. One example is The Kyoto Protocol, an agreement between countries ensuring a reduction in carbon dioxide emissions. Concerns over the safety of our food supply and availability of healthy foods has been prompted the U.S. Federal Drug Agency (FDA) and the Federal Government to increase funding and manpower to improve the quality of our food supply. The FDA has also expanded its involvement of regulation of medical radiation exposure, the most common source of harmful radiation. Due to the increase in adverse effects from radiation exposure (hair loss, skin changes, etc.), the FDA is mandating improvements in quality assurance practices, closer monitoring of devices and radiation doses to which patients are exposed, and the development of national registries for radiation doses.

Large scale changes may take several years to come to fruition. But, you can take steps now to reduce your exposure to environmental stress. You can choose where you live, how you live, what you eat and drink, and how loud you like your music.

STRESS AND RELATIONSHIPS

While being involved in a loving, trusting and honest relationships can provide a huge range of benefits – from better sleep to better skin, the flip side of intimacy means that when love or friendship have "gone south" your health and happiness suffer.

It is likely not coincidental that the list of most stressful professions and the list of professions with the highest divorce rates overlap considerably. These professions include: politicians, taxi cab drivers, police officers, fire fighters, and doctors. Time away from family and **stress levels beyond what is considered normal** are most often to blame.

If you want to talk about stress as it relates to work AND family, a group particularly affected by stress-induced divorce are members of the armed forces. A 2009 report released by the Pentagon found the divorce rate of all divisions of the armed services to be on the rise. Quoting Joe Davis, a spokesman for the Veterans of Foreign Wars, "Every marriage has controllable and uncontrollable factors, but when you interject eight years of war, preparing for war, being at war, coming home and having to think about going back to war again - and when you have children - it just has a tremendous impact on the family unit." And don't forget the stress of war manifests in several types of mental health conditions, including PTSD, a condition strongly associated with low cortisol states as we will discuss further in Chapter Eight.

With respect to divorce, stress is at the top of the list of causes. In the U.S., the divorce rates for first, second, and third marriages are 41 percent, 60 percent, and 73 percent respectively.

Our stress also affects how we relate to our children. Consider how you feel when you come home from a long day at the office. You are mentally and emotionally spent and are wondering how you are going to muster the enthusiasm to cook dinner, help your child complete her homework, and somehow manage to fit in some "quality time" (and perhaps extra work!) before bedtime.

Although it is unimaginable for most of us to think about abusing or neglecting our children, stress can both impair our mental and emotional health and also lead us to take on negative habits, like abusing drugs or alcohol. These behaviors can often lead to neglect of self and children. A 2004 report released by the *National Institute of Justice* found there to be a direct correlation between stress and domestic violence. The report cited such stressors as spousal unemployment and couples under financial strain to result in rates of abuse three times higher than in the general population.

Stress on today's working families is further fueled by the very limited access to quality daycare. Further, family members nowadays may be scattered across the globe leaving many parents without the help of grandparents or other relatives to assist with child-rearing and emotional support. This puts further stress on duel and single parents who are then 100 percent responsible for all things emotional, physical and material when it comes to child-rearing. If it takes a village to raise a child, than we better start developing a new urban plan - quick.

Having had the chance to delve into the details surrounding environmental, societal and work-related stress, you may feel overwhelmed. Luckily, in democratic countries such as ours, we're free to explore new work opportunities, new relationships and new experiences. Our lives will clearly never permit us to avoid *everything* potentially toxic to our stress response systems. By improving personal habits and choices, engaging in community outreach and education, and helping to amplify the voices of law-makers and organizations who promote healthy environments, you can join others in fueling the winds of change.

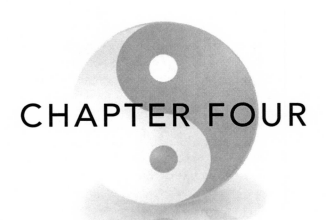

CHAPTER FOUR

Decoding The Truth: Moving Beyond "Adrenal Fatigue"

"He who has health, has hope; and he who has hope, has everything."

Arabian Proverb

In Chapter One, I touched on my reservations about "adrenal fatigue." And, while I'm wary of belaboring the point, the sub-title of this book is, after all, "outsmarting stress" and, in order to outsmart stress, we need to fully understand the hard science about how our bodies really work. In this vein, the topic merits a much more detailed discussion of the adrenal fatigue phenomenon. In fact, this entire chapter is dedicated to exploring it further.

To give you a taste of the growing concern in the scientific field about the issue, I was recently quoted in a blog post for *Ortho-Molecular Products* contemplating, "Is Adrenal Fatigue just a Phantom 'Internet Disease'?" Here's an excerpt from that article and my response to it:

In August 2010, *the Hormone Foundation and Endocrine Society* published

LENA D. EDWARDS MD, FAARM

and distributed their "Myth vs. Fact" sheet about Adrenal Fatigue where they claim:

"Adrenal fatigue is not a real medical condition. There are no scientific facts to support the theory that long-term mental, emotional, or physical stress drains the adrenal glands and causes many common symptoms. There is no test that can detect adrenal fatigue. Supplements and vitamins made to "treat" adrenal fatigue may not be safe. Taking these supplements when you don't need them can cause your adrenal glands to stop working and may put your life in danger."

My Response:

"There is absolutely no dispute within the medical literature, which spans almost eighty years, on the effects of both acute and chronic stress on aging, disease formation, and early mortality. And though it is true the science does not validate the existence of primary adrenal gland failure independent of all other organ systems, the use of the term 'adrenal fatigue' has been beneficial in promoting the recognition of the relationship between stress and disease. Unfortunately, the use of this term has been detrimental in several respects.

First of all, the adrenal glands are just one of many organs and structures involved in the stress response system. And as members of a system, they *cannot* and *do not* act independently. To promote the adrenal gland as being an independently functioning, central component of the stress response system is not only inaccurate but also diminishes the true complexity of the neuroendocrinological system."

If you're keen to know how followers of adrenal fatigue classify the disorder, here is a short definition: A maladaptive state in which adrenal corticosteroid production is significantly diminished in response to repetitive and chronic psychological stress; the resulting state of hypoadrenia then renders the body incapable of:

- Perpetuating an adaptive chronic fight or flight response
- Mounting an appropriate stress response to acute stressors
- "Adrenals simply cannot keep up with demands placed upon them"

So, if adrenal fatigue is not accurate or useful, what do healthcare providers, whether conventional or alternative, have to gain from applying and promoting this diagnosis? Well, it depends. Some may not fully understand the complexities of the stress response system. Others may actually agree with their patients who have self-diagnosed adrenal fatigue or promote this diagnosis in order to promote sales of nutritional supplements to "fix" the problem.

And, yes, there are countless supplements and vitamins available on the market which claim to improve or cure adrenal fatigue. And while many of these supplements are not outrageously expensive (ranging in price from $12 to $50 per bottle), the content, quality, and claims made by some are questionable at best (in light of the lack of FDA regulation). Moreover, some consultants promote an intensive treatment regimen consisting of three or more supplements per day for months or even years. While supplements can be potentially helpful in some patients with low cortisol states and HPA axis (stress system) dysfunction, many patients pay a high price since the cost for "therapy" is often not covered by their health benefit plans. This can be frustrating since some find either partial or no sustained improvement in their symptoms, particularly if the underlying cause of their low cortisol is never identified and treated.

This is not to say that certain pharmaceutical grade supplements have no clinical usefulness. In fact, some have been studied and have been shown to clinically improve dysfunctional stress responses as you will learn later on when we discuss treatment options. Not all supplements are created equal, and I will teach you what to look for.

PRACTICING GOOD MEDICINE

Now that we have a grasp on the pioneering effect that Hans Selye and others had on our comprehension of what stress does to our bodies, we can better appreciate the intricacies of the stress response and why ascribing a "one size fits all" diagnosis of adrenal fatigue to all who are fatigued completely misses the boat.

While the adrenal glands do play a definite role in how we feel day to day (whether that's energetic or exhausted), as we've now established, the term "adrenal fatigue" is, at best, a misnomer. According to the Mayo Clinic (one of several medical establishments in disagreement with this concept), the term adrenal fatigue is used by some practitioners of alternative medicine who claim adrenal fatigue to be too mild to be picked up on standard blood tests. They go on to state that "proponents of this unproven term claim it to be a mild form of adrenal insufficiency rendering a patient incapable of producing enough stress hormones to produce an adequate fight or flight response."

As a physician who has practiced both the traditional [sometimes known as "conventional"] medicine and integrative [inaccurately termed "alternative" or "holistic"] medicine for over a decade, I can tell you that this description ascribed to adrenal fatigue does not adequately describe the complexity of our stress response systems.

Our bodies are quite sophisticated and designed to rebalance or adapt to a variety of assaults. In fact, when we are subjected to either acute or chronic stress, a complex series of events takes place to ensure our survival. Your adrenal glands are only one player in the stress game. And a successful game relies heavily on your adrenals working together with your brain, your immune system, and other systems. To imply that the adrenal glands are central to the entire stress response process and unilaterally responsible for all our undiagnosed symptoms is both short-sighted and inaccurate. To illustrate, here is a snapshot of a relevant case study – a complaint stemming from a patient's encounter with a physician with an interest in holistic medicine –taken from *MD Dialogue* (2008), a newsletter created by the College of Physicians and Surgeons of Ontario:

"On the recommendation of a friend, a female patient decided to see a physician who had an interest in holistic medicine and naturopathic medicine. The patient had a history of fatigue, shortness of breath and frequent colds and wanted to see if complementary medicine could resolve her symptoms... After hearing the patient's history, the doctor diagnosed her as having food allergies, 'tired adrenals,' and an excess amount of yeast in her system...

The doctor believed that the patient's symptom of fatigue, in the presence of low normal cortisol, was consistent with 'adrenal fatigue.' The values of numerous other blood tests also suggested masked food allergies or an imbalance of organisms in the bowel, as possible explanations, she wrote. The doctor recommended Vega testing [a machine that uses low electrical currents to interpret a health profile], specialized blood testing, and advised the patient to purchase certain nutritional supplements...

Overall, the [Complaints] Committee did have some concerns, and decided to require the doctor to be cautioned by a panel of the Complaints Committee. The points of concern were that she should have conducted a physical examination, and she should have been more fulsome in her information provided about Vega testing."

The unfortunate aspect to this scenario is that the patient did have debilitating symptoms, and the physician correctly diagnosed a low cortisol state which appeared to be caused by numerous factors. Unfortunately, the physician partially invalidated her diagnosis and was subsequently penalized by ordering unconventional testing and by not performing a physical examination which is considered to be the "standard of care."

In my experience, this is not uncommon. In fact, some practitioners who diagnose patients with adrenal fatigue are not physicians or qualified healthcare professionals and may not thoroughly understand the proper testing and treatment protocols of low cortisol states. This then contrasts with traditionally trained physicians who learn nothing about how to treat subtle abnormalities in cortisol highs and lows. This not only leaves patients in limbo but also has only served to further fuel the fire of misunderstanding and animosity between the conventional and integrative medical communities.

SEMANTICS MATTER

Why does it matter what term we use to describe how low cortisol states arise? Isn't it just semantics? No! While it's expected and often healthy to have some discord in medicine – it keeps all of us on our toes – there's also a danger when professionals choose to hang on to hypotheses that are no longer valid. Many medical professionals around the world agree

LENA D. EDWARDS MD, FAARM

with my contention that calling this syndrome "adrenal fatigue" is not only misinformed but potentially dangerous as well. It's vitally important to correctly understand how our mind and body function so we can take the proper steps towards corrective action and not neglect potentially serious underlying medical conditions.

I have seen patients who were diagnosed with adrenal fatigue who did have low cortisol, but it wasn't because their adrenals "pooped out." It was actually because they had other underlying diagnoses such as cancer or a chronic infection or a vitamin deficiency, etc. They had seen their doctor or chiropractor or healthcare professional complaining of fatigue, mild depression, and the like, their salivary cortisol levels were low, and they received their 'adrenal fatigue' diagnosis stamp without anyone ever investigating the cause of their low cortisol! In several cancer patients, their adrenal fatigue diagnosis was ultimately their death sentence because, by the time I saw them, it was too late despite the treatment they had received for their adrenal fatigue. For instance, Richard, a sixty-year-old patient later diagnosed with metastatic lung cancer, did not see his doctor at first when he began suffering from extreme fatigue. He did his own research online and discovered a website about adrenal fatigue. After thoroughly reviewing the site and deciding he could have offered his services as the poster child given the dramatic overlap of his symptoms, he promptly ordered ten different "adrenal boosting" supplements. After six months of taking these supplements and finding they were not helping, he finally decided to see his doctor... and by that time, it was too late.

If you have already been diagnosed with or think you may have adrenal fatigue or you're just learning about the dispute behind the adrenal fatigue diagnosis, this is a lot to take in. So, if you feel frustrated, please don't. The good news is that you've taken the first steps in better understanding stress and how it can either help you in the short term or make you feel bad and potentially even get sick if it is chronic in nature. Reading *Adrenalogic* takes this a step further by empowering you with even more knowledge so that you are not misdiagnosed and thus mistreated – you can take control of you. Being told you have adrenal fatigue is like being told you have a fever. The question you will now become proficient in asking your doctor is: "Why?!"

LEGITIMIZING YOUR DIAGNOSIS:
THE CURRENT CONSENSUS

To further emphasize the need for a change in terminology and how semantics truly are standing in the way of medical progress and understanding, here is a small sampling of feedback from a variety of well-respected and widely reviewed medical organizations.

"Adrenal fatigue" is not a real medical condition. There are no scientific facts to support the theory that long-term mental, emotional, or physical stress drains the adrenal glands and causes many common symptoms... Supplements and vitamins made to "treat" adrenal fatigue may not be safe. Taking these supplements when you don't need them can cause your adrenal glands to stop working and may put your life in danger."

From the Endocrine Society web site, Chevy Chase, MD

"There's no question that fatigue is at least partly due to the interactions between the brain and the adrenal glands. But it's a gross oversimplification of the origins of fatigue to imply that the adrenals are a major cause."

Dr. Daniel Clauw, Director of Chronic Pain & Research Center, University of Michigan

"Adrenal fatigue is a worthless diagnosis... claims of marked improvement following some intervention most likely fraudulent."

Dr. Paul Rosch, President American. Institute of Stress

"Is adrenal fatigue real? Yes and no... Like many things in this arena, it's a grain of truth surrounded by a lot of hype and peddlers of quick fixes."

Dr. Brent Bauer, Mayo Clinic Complementary and Integrative Medicine Program

"Proponents of adrenal fatigue claim that it's caused by chronic stress. There also are claims that special tests, available for purchase, are needed to diagnose adrenal fatigue. By seeking unproven tests or treatments for adrenal fatigue, you could delay the diagnosis of a real, treatable

condition or take something that would impair the adrenal glands. Adrenal supplements, sold in stores or on the Internet, can suppress the amount of hormones produced by the adrenal glands. Patients dealing with extreme fatigue or who suspect an adrenal problem should seek care from an internist or primary care physician. A doctor can also look for other problems that could be the underlying cause of fatigue or muscle aching, such as depression, fibromyalgia and obstructive sleep apnea."

"It's frustrating to have persistent symptoms your doctor can't readily explain. But accepting a medically unrecognized diagnosis from an unqualified practitioner could be worse. Unproven remedies for so-called "adrenal fatigue" may leave you feeling sicker, while the real cause — such as depression or fibromyalgia — continues to take its toll."

Todd Nippoldt, MD, Endocrinologist at the Mayo Clinic. (Mayoclinic.com)

The simplistic nature of this label truly underestimates the complexity of the mind-body connection and undermines our body's capacity to persevere in the face of chronic stress. In addition, the term is an unrecognized medical diagnosis within the traditional medical community bringing only mockery and disappointment to any patient presenting to their physician with a self-affixed diagnosis of adrenal fatigue. I suggest, as do many of my colleagues, that we use the long-standing term "HPA axis dysfunction" when referring to the actual cause of stress-related disorders and diseases influenced by the HPA axis. Furthermore, conditions of abnormally low cortisol (whether chronically low or abnormally low in response to an acute stress) are more accurately termed **hypocortisolism**, not adrenal fatigue.

BEYOND ADRENAL FATIGUE: DYSFUNCTION VS. DISEASE

Now, I'm not going to tell you that the symptoms of the millions of people (perhaps you!) diagnosed with adrenal fatigue are not real. In fact, a huge number of my own patients come to me describing symptoms of:

- General exhaustion and fatigue
- Foggy thinking and difficulty concentrating

- Depression
- Chronic pain syndromes (i.e. fibromyalgia)
- Difficulty sleeping
- Intolerance to stress

However, though these symptoms are real and do derive in part from adrenal *gland dysfunction*. I must reiterate what I said in the initial article excerpt: the adrenal glands cannot and do not act independently. You see, it's the HPA axis: hypothalamus + pituitary gland + adrenal glands (illustrated below). The HPA axis is then influenced by numerous other hormones and organ systems which ultimately culminates in the function or dysfunction I discuss in this book.

To use an analogy, it's kind of like a football team. The quarterback does not make all of the plays and act independently of his team; he strategizes, discusses the plays with his team-mates who then signal each other to carry out the action. The strongly influential crowd in the background then subliminally affects the team by either cheering them to victory or booing them to defeat. That's hard science – and it's good sportsmanship!

LOCATION OF THE COMPONENTS OF THE HYPOTHALAMIC-PITUITARY-ADRENAL (HPA) AXIS

the body's stress-response football team

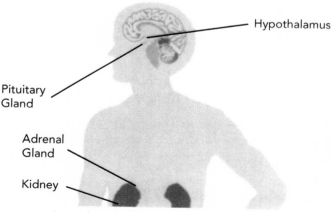

Image from the National Institute of Health

LENA D. EDWARDS MD, FAARM

While the symptoms listed above are common, they are generally not life-threatening and thus often missed by traditional testing methods. However, there are two rare but serious diseases associated with dysfunctional adrenal glands – Cushing's Syndrome and Addison's Disease.

Cushing's Syndrome occurs as the result of too much cortisol in the blood for an extended period of time. The two types of Cushing's Syndrome, exogenous (from an outside source) and endogenous (from a source within the body), share a common list of symptoms but different causes. Exogenous Cushing's Syndrome occurs in patients taking cortisol-like medications, and is temporary, ceasing when the patient has finished the course of medication. The endogenous form of this endocrine system disease is far rarer, and results from a tumor or tumors either on the adrenal glands or the pituitary gland.

Cushing's Syndrome symptoms include the following:
- Weight gain
- Bone loss
- Muscle loss and weakness
- Easily-bruised, fragile skin
- Reduced sex drive
- Menstrual disturbances
- Depression/inability to think clearly

Addison's Disease, also among the rare endocrine system diseases, occurs in fewer than one hundred and fifty people in a million. Also referred to as primary adrenal insufficiency, Addison's Disease occurs when the adrenal glands produce an insufficient amount of steroid hormones despite the presence of an adequate amount of ACTH, the hormone that triggers the adrenal glands to release steroids. Most often, this condition occurs as a result of actual destruction of adrenal gland tissue either from infections or from autoimmune disease.

The steroid hormones produced by the adrenal glands, and deficient during Addison's Disease, hold many important functions including the regulation of blood sugar levels, helping the body fight infection and stress, and maintaining normal sexual drive.

Addison's Disease symptoms include the following:

- Fatigue, weakness, loss of appetite
- Muscle and joint pain
- Gastrointestinal problems (nausea, vomiting, etc.)
- Darkening of the skin on the face, neck, and back of hands
- Low blood pressure and blood sugar
- A craving for salt

It is interesting to note that many patients with low (but not absent) cortisol have many of the same symptoms as patients with Addison's Disease, albeit more mild in nature. In fact, Dr. Baschetti has written numerous articles astutely pointing out that patients with chronic fatigue syndrome, a condition associated with hypocortisolism, share forty-three symptoms with patients who have Addison's Disease. He goes so far as to propose that chronic fatigue syndrome be termed "sub-clinical Addison's Disease." I will elaborate on this further when we discuss hypocortisolism in Chapter Eight.

STRESSORS AND THE HPA AXIS: WHY, WHAT, AND HOW

Stressors go beyond where you work or who you are married to. In fact, anything your body perceives as disrupting internal balance, whether internal or external, is considered a stressor. It is also interesting to note that not all stressors are created equal. Whether and to what extent a stressor is perceived as stressful is influenced by different aspects not only of the individual person but also of the stressor. With respect to any situation or event, there are distinct qualities that will define if that event is perceived as stressful or not.

Here are some examples of stressors that can cause HPA axis dysfunction and abnormal cortisol states (which will be discussed in more detail later):

- Adrenal injury (trauma, haemorrhage, auto-immune diseases)
- Brain or spinal cord injury
- Drug directly toxic to the adrenal glands (certain drugs)
- Nearly all over the counter or prescription medications

- Nutritional deficiencies (i.e. B1, B5, Vitamin C)
- Deficiencies of materials required for cortisol production (progesterone, HDL cholesterol)
- Chronic diseases (i.e. diabetes, heart disease)
- Exposures to chemicals, pollution, and radiation (i.e. in our food and our environment)
- Food allergies
- Psychological stress
- Heavy metal toxicity
- Viral, bacterial, and fungal infections
- "Leaky gut" (unhealthy digestive tract)

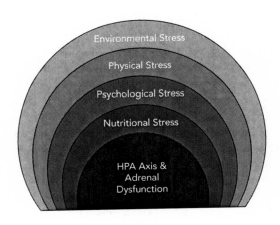

When we are speaking of psychological stressors in particular, there is yet another layer of complexity in defining if and to what extent our HPA axis is disturbed. This aspect revolves around us as individuals — how old we are, our gender, our lifetime experiences, and our personalities. You may not think that what happened to you years ago when you were in your mother's womb or when you were growing up as a child would affect your body's stress response system once you are an adult, but in fact it does! As we touched on earlier in this book, research has shown that your stress response system may have been damaged early on in your life if your mother used drugs or alcohol or if she had chronic health problems during her pregnancy.

During childhood, such factors as psychological or sexual abuse or abandonment may also have left permanent scars on the HPA axis. If you are older or if you are female, your stress response is also more likely to be abnormal. Finally, your personality characteristics are very important in determining how you respond to stress. People who are "Type A" personalities, or are easily angered, competitive, introverted, or 'control freaks' are also more likely to have HPA axis dysfunction and unhealthy responses to stress. Clearly, it makes sense that those of us 'high strung' people are more likely to get excited about things causing our HPA axis to be activated and our cortisol levels to go up. It's ironic, but if our stress response systems stay on hyper-drive long enough and low cortisol then develops, our fuses become even shorter and we are more likely to react and less likely to recover from additional stress.

As an example of how one's personality and outlook affect stress and therefore health, I once had two patients, "Joanne" and "Kim," who were friends and worked in the same office. They were both in their mid-thirties and had two small children. Joanne was very upbeat. She exercised, ate healthy food, and most importantly, she had a very optimistic outlook. Joanne was laid back and took life as it came. The other patient, Kim, was exactly the opposite. She was very controlling, a perfectionist, and tended to be a "glass half empty" kind of person.

Because of these dissimilar personality traits, the two patients' salivary cortisol patterns were completely different even though so many aspects of their lives were the same. Joanne had a seemingly normal cortisol curve while Kim had an abnormal salivary cortisol pattern: low during the day and paradoxically high in the evening. Kim later developed high blood sugar, high blood pressure, and obesity – ultimately requiring prescription medication. Joanne, on the other hand, enjoyed spending her extra cash on vacations instead of prescription drugs.

DISCONNECTION CAN CAUSE DYSFUNCTION

As we have already discussed, the HPA axis is made of many players and these players are influenced by other factors like the immune system, hormones, neurotransmitters, etc. So if we again use the analogy of the

LENA D. EDWARDS MD, FAARM

football game, you can more easily understand how things can go awry. Perhaps the quarterback gives the order for the next play but the players do not listen. Alternatively, the quarterback may neglect to give any strategic orders at all. The plan may be carried out to perfection, but the football doesn't make it over the goal line (cortisol cannot work or get into cells). If the quarterback or any of the players are injured (by the stressors mentioned above) that will also affect their ability to play effectively if at all.

Then there is the influence of the crowd (immune system, neuroendocrine system, etc.) indirectly influencing the players on the team. The crowd can cheer (up-regulate), boo (down-regulate), or tell the players to run in the wrong direction. If it then rains on the crowd, their reactions may be influenced even further. We haven't even mentioned the home life of the players, the role their parents and siblings play in affecting their behavior, morale, and motivation. All of these influences, whether direct or indirect, can ultimately result in a successful play and therefore a touchdown. If the football does not cross the line (hypocortisolism), you can now see how many different places the disconnect can occur!

To further add to this already overwhelmingly complex picture, here is just one more thing to consider on this subject: In some patients, low cortisol is actually considered a *normal variant*, meaning that the person is not suffering any symptoms at all even though their cortisol levels are sub-par. In others, low cortisol becomes their new set point after exposure to chronic stress. As we learned on Day One of medical school... *treat the patients, not the numbers!* Or, as we mentioned in Chapter Three, "all stress is not created equal." Now that you have a better understanding of *what* causes low cortisol states, *where* do you look to find and treat this problem? Read on to quench the suspense...

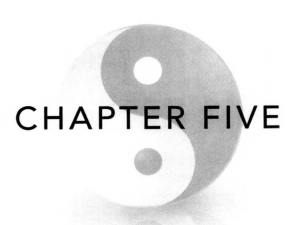

CHAPTER FIVE

Where To Look: Identifying and Diagnosing Abnormal Cortisol Levels

The more original a discovery, the more obvious it seems afterwards.

Arthur Koestler

At this point in *Adrenalogic*, we've had the chance to dissect the inner workings of the stress response system, and fully appreciate how stress affects our health, our longevity, and society at large. So in order to identify the appropriate solutions, you must first identify from whence the abnormalities originate. In this chapter, I review the different types of testing available to assist you and your healthcare provider in accurately assessing underlying stress hormone levels.

Researchers and physicians determine cortisol levels through three main bodily fluids: <u>saliva, blood, and urine. Hair analysis for cortisol levels is also on the horizon</u>. We will discuss some of these in detail, including the pros, cons, and factors that can influence how test results are interpreted.

BLOOD (SERUM) TESTING

Historically, serum testing has been the tried and true test to assess cortisol levels. Serum represents the watery fraction of your blood that has already passed through your tissues, meaning that all nutrients and hormones have been extracted. It is also void of red blood cells which are major carriers of many substances, including hormones. As is true of urine testing, serum testing for cortisol levels is specifically designed to pick up abnormalities *only if they are outside the laboratory's normal reference range*. And herein lays problem number one:

Reference ranges in labs for all tests are statistically derived and not based on optimal physiological function. Typically, the reference is a set range wherein 95 percent of the population should fall. In contrast, optimal range is a limit that is based on serum levels associated with optimal health or levels associated with a decreased risk of acquiring a disease.

Thus, when your doctor tells you that all of your blood tests are "in the normal range," she is telling you that you are statistically the same as 95 percent of the population. Unfortunately, the population used to establish the reference range has not been screened to ensure they are optimally healthy. Furthermore, references range may vary with age, sex, race, diet, use of prescribed or herbal drugs and stress. Reference ranges also vary from one lab to another and can be affected by different chemical substances used by different labs; this happens with cortisol testing as well. There are several obvious drawbacks to checking cortisol using serum alone. First of all, within the first hour of awakening, cortisol levels fluctuate considerably. So, depending upon when you have your lab work done, it may appear too high or too low since a single blood draw cannot give an average. Secondly, for a true assessment and more important than the first morning cortisol level, is the *pattern* of cortisol secretion during the course of the day. To determine this accurately, four blood draws spaced four to five hours apart are required – this is most certainly impractical and inconvenient! Also, like many other hormones, cortisol "drives" around your blood stream stuck to a protein called *cortisol binding globulin*. You might want to imagine it kind of like a traffic jam: The more cars on the highway (higher levels of binding protein), means the more people can get into these cars (cortisol is more bound or stuck). If fewer people are available because they are stuck in traffic (less free cortisol), the less available they will be to work.

We haven't even mentioned the not so obvious disadvantages like the pain of having a needle stuck in your arm or the traffic you had to fight to get to the lab. Both of these (and other) stressors will falsely elevate what your true morning cortisol may actually be. For instance, I once had a patient who had symptoms of low morning cortisol, but her morning serum cortisol was always elevated. Upon further questioning, she told me she had a crush on the lab technician that was drawing her blood work, and she was always nervous when she saw him!

In general, serum testing for cortisol tends to overestimate true underlying cortisol levels (in some cases by up to 70 percent). An excellent article published by Dr. Holtorf (*Journal of Chronic Fatigue*, 2008) discusses not only the overall inaccuracy but also the marked variation in test results depending upon the components used by the laboratory.

"It has been shown that the plasma cortisol immunoassays used by the majority of laboratories, institutions, and studies suffer from considerable inaccuracy and variance and can significantly overestimate serum cortisol levels when compared to gold standards... This has led to controversy, a high degree of misdiagnosis and the misclassification of patients as having normal HPA function despite significant dysfunction or severely underestimating the severity of the dysfunction."

There are also other types of serum testing known as stimulation tests or suppression tests whereby someone with abnormally low or high cortisol levels is given a medication to induce a given response. Again, these tests are specifically designed to detect Addison's Disease or Cushing's Disease and may completely miss 95 percent of the population in the "normal reference range" who have subtle abnormalities in stress hormone levels.

URINE TESTING

Urine testing (over twenty-four hours) is also used to assess cortisol levels in patients; it offers several obvious advantages. One is that the patient can avoid a needle stick by collecting their own urine at home. It also allows an estimate of what a person's cortisol levels are over a twenty-four hour period. In addition, it's useful in determining how your body is using or 'metabolizing' cortisol since cortisol's by-products are eliminated in the urine. This test has been traditionally used as a gold standard in diagnosing patients with Cushing's Disease.

Urine testing does carry some drawbacks, however, a major problem being errors in collection of the urine (I have seen some very interesting results in this regard!). Also, like serum testing, urine testing does not allow for your doctor to see how your cortisol levels change over the course of the day: the pattern is key. As well, there are large variations in how your body eliminates cortisol in the urine, and in general, urine testing has been shown in some studies to *underestimate* true levels (by up to 30 percent).

My preference when testing patients? I find a twenty-four-hour urine collection for free cortisol levels to be useful in patients who are unable to collect saliva samples or in patients whose daytime salivary cortisol levels are very low or "flat" I often find that patients who have flattened daytime cortisol patterns may be making their cortisol at night instead of during the day (as is the case in insomniacs). A test result like that – in central or upper part of the reference range – helps to guide me in determining what is going on in the middle of the night when the patient is sleeping and not spitting into a test tube.

SALIVARY TESTING

Saliva testing of steroid (cortisol and other) hormones has been documented in the medical literature for nearly thirty years. In fact, measurement of salivary cortisol specifically has been standard medical practice for more than twenty years. In the 1990's, the World Health Organization approved this method of testing as an accurate and convenient way to check free hormone levels. Although used mainly for research purposes at first, saliva testing has gained distinctive diagnostic credibility not only in assessing stress hormone levels but also in testing for infectious diseases, food allergies, certain cancers, and other medical conditions.

WHY SALIVA?

As we have already discussed, one of the shortcomings of serum testing is that hormones circulate stuck to protein "cars" and as such, this makes them unavailable to do their jobs in the tissues. In simple terms, the bio-available fraction of the hormones represents what our cells are actually able to use. Assessing hormones in the saliva bypasses this problem because technically, saliva is tissue. Since binding proteins (cars) are not necessary for hormones (people) to exist in saliva, they exist in their free or "bio-available" form and so can be reliably measured.

Saliva testing offers several advantages to other traditional forms of testing:

- Stress-free collection method
- Non-invasive (no needles)
- Convenient and cost effective
- Does not require special processing
- Represents the free or bio-available fraction of hormones
- Allows for examination of the pattern or diurnal variation of cortisol release
- Allows for evaluation of influential lifestyle factors on an individual's cortisol release
- Collections over multiple days allows for evaluation of cyclic variations in cortisol release
- Samples stable for several weeks without requiring processing or freezing

Although not yet considered the gold standard for testing, saliva is still widely utilized by practitioners to determine levels of both the sex hormones (progesterone, estrogen, and testosterone) and stress hormones (cortisol and DHEA). In fact, in 2008 the *Endocrine Society Clinical Practice Guidelines* endorsed midnight salivary cortisol testing as an appropriate tool in diagnosing patients with Cushing's Disease. Below are some examples of typical salivary cortisol release patterns.

LENA D. EDWARDS MD, FAARM

NORMAL SALIVARY CORTISOL PATTERN

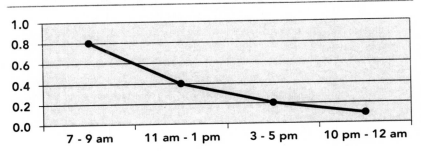

Figure 1: Normal salivary cortisol release pattern measured in mcg/dL

This is Frank's cortisol pattern results. Frank is a thirty-eight-year-old banker whose main complaint was depression. He also had some anxiety, insomnia, and foggy thinking. Frank's depression had started five years earlier and the several medications he tried did not help. He was asked to collect his saliva during a typical work day.

HYPERCORTISOLISM CURVE

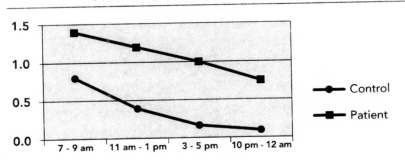

These are the results from Susan's testing. Susan is a fifty-year-old high school teacher who had been diagnosed with fibromyalgia by her doctor.

Despite every medication she tried, she continued to "hurt all over." Her lab tests were always "in the normal range." Susan had tried a number of over-the-counter supplements which were marginally helpful. Her pain was always worse on week days and so that is when she collected her saliva samples.

HYPERCORTISOLISM CURVE

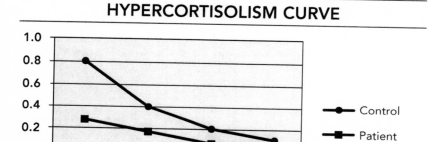

ALL THAT IS FLAT IS NOT "FATIGUED"

So you go to your doctor to review the results of your tests which reveal you have a flattened (very low) daytime cortisol pattern. Eureka! Adrenal fatigue, right? NOT! Indeed, even though salivary cortisol patterns are very helpful in determining the healthiness of your HPA axis and functionality of your stress response system, there are many hidden factors that can taint the picture taken in that twenty-four-hour snapshot.

Studies have actually revealed significant individual variation in salivary cortisol patterns. These factors include such things as genetics, gender, medications, lifestyle choices, and even time of the year the saliva is collected. In general, men tend to have a more heightened cortisol than women because their adrenal glands are more responsive to stress in general. In fact some studies have shown that even the *anticipation* of forthcoming stress causes a male's salivary cortisol levels to rise. Women may be surprised to know that if they collect their saliva during the first part of their menstrual cycle (commonly known as the *follicular phase*) or take oral contraceptives, their salivary cortisol levels may be significantly flattened.

Things get even more interesting when you factor in the bad habits we acquire to combat stress. Nicotine, as one example, is a potent stimulator of our stress response systems. However, regular consumption from nicotine reduces the ability of the stress system to respond to the repeated onslaught of acute stressors and blunts salivary cortisol release patterns.

Most of us have also developed a passionate love affair with coffee because of the cortisol stimulating of caffeine. Unfortunately, as is true with everything else in life: too much + too long = too bad. When chronically consumed, cortisol responses to caffeine are ultimately reduced. Those of you who eat carbohydrate laden breakfast cereals every morning may as well hang it up also. Alcohol is another security blanket we wrap around our stress. Unfortunately, chronic alcohol consumption and even acute alcohol intake can impact the salivary responses to acute stressors.

And then there are the drugs and supplements we take. *Nearly every single medication, including over-the-counter medications, can directly or indirectly affect salivary cortisol release patterns.* To list them all would require a separate book in and of itself, so I will provide you with a list of some of the more commonly medications that can affect your otherwise naive salivary cortisol pattern:

- Corticosteroids (oral, nasal, topical, inhaled)
- Cardiovascular medications (drugs for high blood pressure, high cholesterol, heart failure, heart arrhythmia)
- Psychotropics (sleeping pills, anti-depressants, anti-psychotics, anti-anxiety medications)
- Oral contraceptives and other hormones
- Anti-cholinergic drugs (such as drugs to treat over active bladder, irritable bowel syndrome, and asthma)
- Pain medications (i.e. narcotics/opioids, tylenol, anti-inflammatory medications, muscle relaxants)

Finally, believe it or not, some people simply do not have the expected normal pattern of cortisol release and *it does not cause any problems...*

Flat without fatigue. In fact, some studies have found that among randomly selected individuals, 10 to 15 percent did not show the typical diurnal or circadian pattern of cortisol release. This is yet another reminder that all human beings are unique and that "one size does not fit all" when it comes to treatment for stress-related diseases or any other disorders for that matter.

THE CORTISOL AWAKENING RESPONSE (CAR)

The CAR or *cortisol awakening response* deserves brief but special mention because it can mean something very important. As we have repeatedly discussed, cortisol is released in a typical diurnal pattern. The highest cortisol levels occur in the second half of the night and peak in the early morning hours coinciding with when we wake up. In the first twenty to thirty minutes after we awake in the morning, there is a very rapid rise in cortisol levels called the CAR. Interestingly, this same CAR does not occur if we wake up in the middle of the night or from a daytime nap.

Studies have shown that the very first morning saliva collection can be a big clue as to the functionality of your stress response system and specifically, the responsiveness of your adrenal glands to the stress message they receive from your brain. So, if you have a saliva test and your morning cortisol level is normal or high, then your adrenal glands are following commands normally. If your first cortisol level is low, then something is interfering with the message the brain is sending to the adrenal glands.

Abnormal CARs can help your doctor hone in on potential causes of your dysfunctional stress response system.

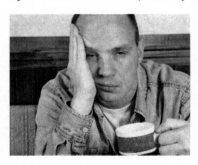

Low CAR has been associated with:

- Metabolic syndrome
- Medication influence (from drugs taken at bedtime)
- Certain mood disorders
- Low socioeconomic status

LENA D. EDWARDS MD, FAARM

High CAR has been associated with:

- Chronic stress and worrying
- Work overload
- Social stress
- Lack of social recognition
- Increased stress early in the day
- Anticipation of upcoming daily demands

Becoming aware of the various methods used to assess cortisol patterns – with salivary being the optimal method - and what can be determined from them means that you have a much better grasp of what cortisol levels represent. You also now know that some people have unusual levels of cortisol but that doesn't mean they're unhealthy – like so many other things in biology, it's just a quirk of nature. With this knowledge in hand, we move on to explore cortisol's relationship with other hormones in our body.

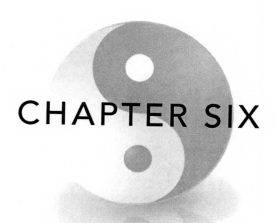

CHAPTER SIX

Communication: Understanding the Synergy Between Hormones

"No one can whistle a symphony.
It takes a whole orchestra to play it. "

H.E. Luccock

In the last chapter, we went over the potential causes of abnormal cortisol levels and release patterns, the different methods used in collection and assessment, and what an imbalance might signify. We now know that the hormone cortisol is critically important to the stress response system. But, let's not forget the other human hormones which, in conjunction with cortisol, control aspects of our stress, growth, sexuality, aging and reproduction. Your hormones harmonize together much like a symphony. To disregard the interactions and interrelationships between hormones would be akin to playing Beethoven's fifth movement without the string section.

Cortisol is your body's primary **catabolic** or "wear and tear" hormone. As we have already discussed, it is also the hormone responsible for providing you with the fuel you need to escape your assailant or fight the bully on the

LENA D. EDWARDS MD, FAARM

playground. By necessity, this fuel is acquired from the breakdown of bone, muscles, and other tissues if necessary.

The remaining hormones, such as estrogen, progesterone, testosterone, insulin, and growth hormone, are all **anabolic hormones** or "growth and repair" hormones. Their actions on bones, muscles, and other tissues are opposite that of cortisol – they repair instead of tear down. **Understanding this basic physiology should make it much easier for you to understand how cortisol interacts with other hormones under the influence of chronic stress.**

To fully understand the synergy of the human hormones in relation to our stress response system, let's use the analogy of a cocktail party:

Cortisol is the VIP at the latest hot party. Other guests (hormones like estrogen, progesterone and DHEA) arrive at the bash and interact with cortisol in various ways—greeting it, scoffing at it, talking badly behind its back, or ignoring it. As the VIP, cortisol's presence trumps that of all the other hormones so it doesn't particularly care about the antics of these "less important" guests. During these interactions, and depending on the levels and functions of these other hormones, the party can turn out to be a raging success or easily get out of hand, depending upon whether cortisol keeps its cool or turns into a drunk raving lunatic. You see, when **cortisol is out of whack, everything else at the "hip, hormone bash" (our bodies) is affected too!**

The relationships between cortisol and the other "hormone party-goers" will be better understood if we introduce and identify the key members of the guest list. Keep in mind that all hormones are the same in both men and women – they merely differ in amount and function.

KEY HORMONES

ALDOSTERONE

Aldosterone is produced by the adrenal glands in response to stress, potassium and sodium levels, and fluid balance. Its job is to make sure that blood pressure, sodium levels, and potassium levels stay stable. For those of you who have low blood pressure, get lightheaded when you try to get up, have occasional heart palpitations, or crave salt, you may consider asking your doctor to check your aldosterone levels.

Like cortisol, aldosterone is released in response to ACTH (or adrenocorticotropic hormone) so certain patients with low cortisol may inevitably have low aldosterone if the problem is stemming from the command center of the stress response system (hypothalamus or pituitary gland both located in the brain).

ESTROGEN

Estrogen is an extremely important hormone in both men and women, controlling hundreds of functions throughout the body. Although we often identify estrogen as a female hormone of reproduction and sexual characteristics, estrogen is also important in maintaining a healthy heart and blood vessels, brain, bones, lungs, and intestinal tract, in addition to affecting both libido (sex drive), and mood.

Many women are concerned about estrogen supplementation because of its potential to induce breast cancer. Certainly, this is a concern and one which has been substantiated by studies using oral synthetic estrogens, *particularly when they are combined with oral progestins (NOT progesterone)*. However, when we consider the protective functions of our own innate estrogen, we find that **the number one risk factor for breast cancer is actually advanced age**; and this happens when estrogen levels have declined.

Indeed, **today's *number one* killer of American women is cardiovascular disease, not breast cancer**. Contemplate the data emerging from years of medical research demonstrating how estrogen reduces the risk of heart disease in a number of different ways:

- Lowers LDL cholesterol
- Improves heart contraction
- Impairs LDL oxidation
- Improves insulin sensitivity
- Lowers lipoprotein (a)
- Lowers blood pressure

ESTROGEN'S EFFECT ON FERTILITY AND MENOPAUSE

LENA D. EDWARDS MD, FAARM

In a premenopausal woman, elevated stress hormones end up "shutting down" estrogen (and progesterone) production on many levels. Additionally, estrogen-sensitive tissues ignore the "hormonal messages" of both estrogen and progesterone, particularly if it is reproductive in nature.

The decrease in estrogen triggered by the increase in cortisol can culminate into such problems as delayed puberty, infertility, and miscarriage. The effect of cortisol on reproduction have clearly been demonstrated in women with Cushing's Disease (hypercortisolism) as evidenced by their lack of ovulation, lack of menses, and infertility.

Interestingly, in aging women, cortisol tends to rise, and is believed this may be partially responsible for postmenopausal women's propensity towards weight gain, mood disorders, inflammation and autoimmune disease, insulin resistance, and increased risk for cardiovascular disease.

TESTOSTERONE

The beneficial roles of testosterone in men (heart, bone, sense of well being, etc.) are equivalent to those of estrogen in women. In men, testosterone is produced in the testes, but in women, both the ovaries and adrenal glands make testosterone. Male sex characteristics, such as facial hair, deep voice, and muscle growth depend upon ample amounts of testosterone. But this hormone is also important in both sexes for maintaining energy levels, sex drive, mood, bones, and mental function.

Perhaps one of testosterone's most important functions in men is to protect the heart. In fact, there is considerable evidence to suggest that **testosterone deficiency** may contribute to the onset, progression, (or both) of cardiovascular disease (CVD). The mechanism through which low testosterone levels contribute to heart disease include increased levels of total and LDL ('bad') cholesterol, increased inflammation, increased thickness of the walls of the arteries, insulin resistance, and endothelial (lining of the blood vessel) dysfunction.

In general, cortisol and testosterone have a "love/hate" relationship. Elevated cortisol can cause reductions in testosterone and vice versa. For example, studies have shown a correlation between elevated levels of testosterone, aggressiveness, and socially delinquent behavior. Presumably because of its testosterone-lowering actions, cortisol has been shown to moderate these and other aggressive behaviors in males with testosterone excess.

PROGESTERONE

Many people think of progesterone as the "pregnancy hormone." However, progesterone is sometimes underappreciated in its ability to affect numerous other physiological processes aside from its function as a reproductive hormone. **Progesterone also plays a critical role as an: anti-inflammatory, anti-muscle spasm, anti-anxiety, and anti-uterine cancer and anti- breast cancer hormone.** Ask any woman who has had a hysterectomy and takes estrogen only as hormone replacement how she feels without progesterone (which is not typically prescribed)... You are likely to get quite an earful!

Another underappreciated function of progesterone is its capacity to function as a neuroprotective hormone, protecting and supporting the brain and therefore improving thought process, focus, and memory. In fact, several studies have found progesterone useful as neuroprotective in patients with brain injuries.

Under normal circumstances, our bodies actually use progesterone to produce cortisol (as well as aldosterone, testosterone, DHEA, and estrogen). And, progesterone levels rise with cortisol in response to stress, in part to serve an anti-inflammatory role. During periods of acute and chronic stress, an interesting phenomenon called "the progesterone steal syndrome" can occur whereby available progesterone is funnelled into cortisol production to meet the increased demand. This can cause a woman to experience low progesterone symptoms such as PMS during periods of stress.

STEROID HORMONE SYNTHESIS PATHWAYS

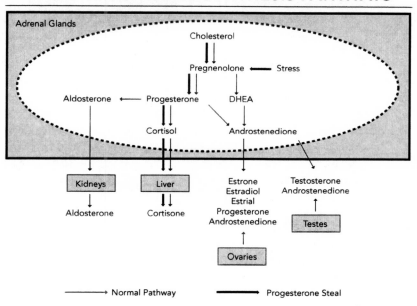

PROLACTIN

Prolactin is produced by the pituitary gland and is primarily involved in the production of breast milk following pregnancy (lactation). However, prolactin is also very important in inhibiting sexual desire (by counteracting dopamine). Prolactin also lowers the levels of estrogen and testosterone. Elevated prolactin levels typically occur because of excessive production by a benign pituitary tumor called a prolactinoma. Symptoms can include inappropriate lactation, lack of menses, loss of underarm and pubic hair, infertility in females and impotence in males.

Stress and cortisol elevations increase prolactin levels. In conjunction with the mayhem that excessive cortisol causes on the reproductive system, cortisol-induced prolactin elevation further suppresses estrogen and progesterone production essentially leaving the reproductive system completely debilitated.

Phew! Are you feeling overwhelmed by all of this data? Let's take a brief break from "Hormones 101" and look at a real world example involving a loving couple who were trying everything (unsuccessfully) to conceive a child.

LANCE AND MAGGIE'S STORY

Maggie was a very determined, sleep-deprived medical resident in her last year of residency when she first came to see me. She had endured her rigorous medical training with pride and integrity intact. Unfortunately, she was much worse for the wear both mentally and physically. Her husband, Lance, was a musician. Their yin-yang personalities and professions made their marriage enviable, so they were both discouraged and frustrated that two years of actively trying to conceive a child had been unsuccessful.

Maggie was only twenty-nine. She and her thirty-two-year-old husband had undergone intensive and expensive fertility testing which yielded "normal" results. No sperm count deficits, no endometriosis or other "female parts" problems, no hormonal deficiencies... *So why?!* Even in vitro fertilization had been unsuccessful three times.

The couple finally came to me as their last hope. Maggie was tearful at the first visit, so Lance did much of the talking.

"Maggie and I are desperate to have a child. All of our friends have kids, and my parents are anxiously awaiting the arrival of a new grandchild. We are trying to do everything we can. We eat only organic foods now, we drink reverse osmosis water, and we try and exercise regularly. For the most part, Maggie tries to stay upbeat about it all, but I know it bothers her because she feels like it is her fault. I keep trying to tell her maybe she just needs to quit stressing about it so much, but I guess that is easier said than done. I just see her changing into another person; her moods are up and down, she tells me that she suffers with PMS, she doesn't sleep well, and she has absolutely no interest in sex."

Maggie sat next to Lance with a forlorn look on her face, nodding in agreement with everything he was saying. So, I started to ask Maggie some initial questions... Questions about her menstrual cycle history,

LENA D. EDWARDS MD, FAARM

questions about her dietary patterns, etc. She had never had any "female problems." She was physically fit on the outside, but as further testing would ultimately reveal, she was a mess on the inside.

I reviewed the results of all testing that had been done, and indeed, everything appeared in the normal range. Thus, problem number one— Maggie was being treated based on her place in the statistically-derived reference ranges of her test results. Actually, many of her hormone levels were on the very low end of the reference range, so they were "normal" but clearly not optimal. Problem number two - at first glance it looked as though no one had checked the status of her HPA axis. Given the fact the cortisol has such a profound influence over production and function of reproductive hormones, it was amazing to me that such a void existed.

Lance agreed with Maggie as she shed additional light on her medical history:

I have been very stressed out since starting medical school seven years ago. I was gone all day long and studied all night long. I seemed better able to handle things at first, maybe because I was younger... I don't know. But as time went by and my work hours got longer, everything seemed to keep getting worse. After I began my medical residency, I was on my feet all day, I would skip meals, and I was on-call a lot. I remember one night, I had fifteen admissions and did not sleep for seventy-two hours. I was exhausted all the time and just kept getting more depressed. Then, I started forgetting things. I even forgot our anniversary a couple of times. I guess at this point, I would settle for just having my life back because I probably would not have the energy to care for a child now anyway."

I explained that **up to 40 percent of couples have no apparent reason for infertility, and it is in this group that researchers believe the effects of stress are most profound.** Interestingly, the rate of unexplained infertility was less than 20 percent two decades ago. Clearly, our bodies have not changed, but our stress levels definitely have!

The reassurance I attempted to provide at their first visit was ultimately trumped by the not so shocking test results providing a probable explanation for why Maggie could not get pregnant. Maggie's stress response system hormones (ACTH, cortisol, and DHEA) were all abnormal. Her salivary cortisol (again, the results from a cortisol test conducted via salivary analysis) showed high cortisol levels throughout the day (which were probably also high at night because she was not sleeping). Basically, Maggie's tissues were "screaming" at the pituitary gland to turn down production of ACTH, the hormone responsible for instructing adrenals to make cortisol. So naturally Maggie's ACTH level was very low. Because her body was in chronic fight or flight mode, the reproductive hormones were being over-powered by the effects of her excessive cortisol.

I explained to Maggie and Lance that **cortisol can cause infertility** by:

1.) "Ordering" the hypothalamus and pituitary gland not to make the hormones that tell the ovaries to make estrogen and progesterone

2.) Shutting down ovarian production of estrogen, progesterone, and testosterone

3.) Commanding the tissues not to listen to progesterone, estrogen, and testosterone even if they are around

4.) Raising prolactin levels which further lowers estrogen and progesterone

Furthermore, excess cortisol negatively affects thyroid hormone (which is defined further down in this chapter) function at multiple levels. And of course, thyroid hormone balance is also essential for normal reproduction. The levels of Maggie's other hormones of growth and repair, namely growth hormone and melatonin, were also low; likely a consequence of both excessive cortisol levels and her lack of sleep since both of these hormones are made at night during sleep (see discussions below). Her DHEA was low which was problematic because its absence allows cortisol levels to rise even higher (since DHEA is the body's natural 'anti-cortisol' hormone). Maggie had also developed numerous nutritional deficiencies from her lack of consistent food intake, and all of those deficiencies were akin to trying to drive a car that has keys in the ignition but no fuel in the tank. Top that off with inflammation and the end result is, well, Maggie.

Given the demands of Maggie's profession, asking her to completely eliminate stress was unrealistic. But, as per my suggestion, she was able to squeeze in ten or fifteen minutes of meditation every night (which has been shown to improve HPA axis function). Short term use of low-dose melatonin at night helped her to sleep which meant over half the battle was already won (since sleep is so vitally important to both reproduction and overall health).

I prescribed phosphatidylserine in divided doses during the day to keep her cortisol levels from going too high, replaced her deficient nutrients by prescribing a specific diet plan and utilizing supplements, and started her on a supplement containing the plant adaptogens Ashwaganda, Maca, Bacopa, and Rhodiola (see Chapter Nine for more details). Instead of skipping meals, she was told to eat small frequent meals throughout the day. She would eat nuts, protein bars, fruits, and vegetables. I also started her on low-dose Naltrexone (See Chapter Nine) to help indirectly combat the inflammation she had as well as to help boost her fertility (as some studies have shown it to do). She also made time to exercise thirty minutes a day four or five times per week.

In three months, Maggie said she felt 50 percent better. In six months, she was 75 percent better. After one year, Maggie called my office in happy tears... "I'm pregnant!" Nine months later, Lance Cole III was born.

And now... Back to our overview of human hormones, Part 2...

DHEA

Also called dehydroepiandrosterone, DHEA is like the party planner for our previously mentioned cocktail party. Without DHEA, cortisol would be allowed to wreak havoc without restraint since **DHEA is your body's main "anti-cortisol" hormone**. But DHEA also does some other very important things:

- Serves as the chief precursor to sex hormones, particularly post-menopause
- Directly binds to receptors in the brain that promote pain relief and relaxation

- Prevents plaque formation ('hardening') of the heart arteries
- Improves insulin sensitivity
- Promotes sense of well being
- Protects the brain
- Maintains tissue strength and repair
- Promotes bone growth
- Enhances immune function in those suffering from autoimmune diseases (particularly rheumatoid arthritis)

But, don't let your excitement over DHEA cause you to go out and buy a big bottle. Even though it is available as an over the counter supplement, its ability to turn into other hormones and lower cortisol warrants extreme caution and medical supervision with its use.

PREGNENOLONE

Pregnenolone is the main conduit between cholesterol and all of the steroid hormones (see graph above). Like DHEA, it is an anti-inflammatory and also antagonizes the effects of cortisol… A party patrol officer if you will. It has also been shown to be of some benefit in maintaining memory as well.

INSULIN

This pancreatic hormone is in charge of regulating the metabolism of carbohydrates (sugars) and fat. It is the hormone responsible for telling your cells to use the fuel (food) you consume for energy. Without insulin, your cells would be in a state of starvation because insulin would not be around to tell them to take up glucose. In the face of chronically elevated cortisol, elevations in blood sugar occur not only because of increased glucose production but also because cells become resistant to the effects of insulin. Consequently, high cortisol states have been associated with the development of Type 2 diabetes as you will read about in Chapter Seven.

GROWTH HORMONE

Growth hormone is another anabolic (growth and repair) hormone produced by the pituitary gland. The highest level of production is during the first hour after we fall asleep. Most adults think growth hormone deficiency means they should be short, but actually, growth hormone serves many important functions in adults including maintenance of muscle, lean body mass, bones, mood, and general health symptoms of growth hormone deficiency include:

- Abdominal obesity
- Muscle wasting
- Bone loss
- Decreased vitality
- Fatigue
- Worsening insulin resistance
- Cardiovascular disease
- Depressed mood

Similar to insulin, cortisol and growth hormone cannot both be the center of attention at the party. This makes sense since when cortisol is around in excessive amounts, growth hormones levels fall - who cares about growth and repair when you are in survival mode, right?

THYROID HORMONE

Thyroid hormone action revs up your system. It's instrumental in the metabolism of protein, carbohydrates, and fats, telling your cells what to do with each type of energy form. Thyroid hormones are also very important in the proper growth and development of cells, long bone development, and neuron (nerve cell) development in the brain. Thyroid hormone ranks second in command after our party VIP, cortisol.

The list of symptoms of low thyroid would fill five pages, but some of the more common ones are:

- Fatigue
- Cold intolerance
- Constipation
- Fluid retention
- Loss of the outer one-third of the eyebrows
- Depression
- Premature aging
- Memory impairment
- Hair loss, dry skin, brittle nails

- Difficulty losing weight/weight retention
- Cholesterol elevation
- Joint and muscle pain
- Slow heart rate
- Menstrual problems and difficulty conceiving

You can imagine what might happen at our party if thyroid decides to take on cortisol. Again, there can't be two VIPs at the party—in other words, if a system is already "revved up" because our VIP, cortisol, is too high, your body will do what it can to prevent spontaneous combustion by inactivating thyroid hormone functions at multiple levels. Not only does cortisol prevent the thyroid gland from getting the message from the brain to make thyroid hormone, it prevents activation of thyroid hormone and renders your cells and tissues insensitive to the actions of thyroid hormone.

Conversely, if a patient with **low cortisol is placed on thyroid hormone, their symptoms may be made much worse.** Why? Because like growth hormone, DHEA, insulin, and pregnenolone, thyroid hormone also antagonizes the effects of cortisol. Think about it this way: since thyroid hormone revs up your system, if cortisol is low, your system cannot be revved up. It would be like trying to enter NASCAR with an empty gas tank.

MELATONIN

Known as "the hormone of darkness," melatonin is released by the pineal gland in the brain. Its primary actions are to help regulate our sleep-wake cycles/circadian rhythms and to serve as a potent anti-oxidant. It can affect reproduction and sex drive by decreasing the levels of the pituitary hormones (FSH and LH) necessary for the production of progesterone, estrogen, and testosterone. **Its effects on the immune system are opposite those of cortisol.** It has been extensively studied and has been shown to have numerous therapeutic implications.

Melatonin has also been shown to reduce cortisol production by inhibiting ACTH, the pituitary hormone that tells your adrenal glands to make cortisol.

LENA D. EDWARDS MD, FAARM

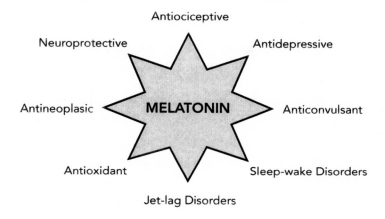

Graph from Rios, ERV, Venancio ET, Rocha, NFM et al. *Melatonin: Pharmacological Aspects and Clinical Trends*; Neuroscience, 120, 583-590, 2010

PUTTING IT ALL TOGETHER

My patient, "Bridget" is a perfect example of someone who had multiple hormone abnormalities from a young age. At mid-life, she had some age-related decline in her sex hormones which were compounded by stress hormone imbalances, and the all-too-common cascade of events stemmed from there...

BRIDGET'S STORY

Bridget was a fiery red head under the rule of her dysfunctional body. When I met her, she was not yet forty-five years old but was already taking several prescription drugs for depression and high blood pressure. She had traveled around the pharmacologic world, trying one anti-depressant medication after another to no avail. The tour had become tiresome and she had run out of destinations. Bridget was near hopeless when I first met her.

Like so many other patients coming to me, Bridget felt as though she was weak and crazy. She had been led to believe that her fatigue, lack of mental clarity, depression, lack of sex drive, weight gain, and sleep disturbances were "all in her head," a statement that was defended by her "normal" test results.

"Over time, my depression got worse. I was in such a fog on some days that I couldn't get out of bed. I missed a lot of work. I managed to stay employed and do okay, although I believe I could have really flourished if I wasn't dealing with the depression. My depression led me to make really bad decisions – a bad marriage for one."

Bridget sought the guidance of various healthcare professionals on her journey to sanity. Unfortunately, no one offered the right solution. Bridget was given one false key to the sanity door after another… Everything from anti-depressants to anti-anxiety medications.

"At age thirty, I could no longer deal with the depression on my own. I finally broke down and saw a psychologist because I was convinced I was going crazy. Despite having a dynamic career as an international tax attorney for a Fortune 500 company, I still had problems getting out of bed and going to work in the morning. I hated my job, my life, my… Everything. My body felt like lead and my head was in a perpetual fog. All I did was crash on the couch after work and sleep on the weekends. I had totally lost all joy in my life."

Bridget's introduction to blood pressure medication came soon after she began taking an anti-depressant.

"I began to wonder why none of these drugs were working on my depression. I developed high blood pressure, dry skin, weight gain, aching joints, a hair trigger temper, digestive trouble, sleep problems and even worse, an inability to concentrate. I saw my primary care physician, who referred me to an endocrinologist about my thyroid. He told me it was "normal" because it fell in the range of "normal" even though it had swollen to the size of a golf ball. I was then sent to a rheumatologist for my aching joints, and was promptly diagnosed with fibromyalgia. I was also referred to a vascular specialist to try to get my blood pressure under control, which was spiking to 180/100 at times. I was also diagnosed with irritable bowel syndrome and basically told to avoid greasy foods. Suddenly, I went from taking one pill to taking six to eight pills a day—yet I still didn't feel any better."

"My caffeine ingestion went through the roof. It was the only thing that got me through each day. I was drinking three to four 20 ounce diet sodas daily just to maintain a decent energy level to get through the day. And I wondered why I had trouble staying asleep at night? I also continued to make irrational decisions.

"At the age of forty, my foggy thinking got worse and the weight gain started in earnest. I am an international tax attorney, which requires me to read detailed tax codes and regulations. I got to the point where I couldn't concentrate anymore to read and digest the new tax laws. I was also forgetting concepts I knew from twenty years ago—basic concepts that I should be able to recall as easily as my name. I couldn't remember names of people I had known for the last twenty years. I was getting scared and panicky. I went another three years just barely hanging on when my hairstylist referred me to Dr. Edwards. My hair was now falling out in gobs. I will always be grateful to her for that referral. It changed my life—the life I never knew could exist. I was at my wits' end when I saw Dr. Edwards. I almost broke down in her office telling her my history. I was hoping she didn't think I was crazy because I was so desperate for someone to help me. I didn't want to live the rest of my life like I had. In fact, if that was all I had to look forward to, I was ready to throw in the towel."

This is a very difficult struggle many patients contend with, especially when they have exhausted all traditional options and truly believe they are banished to such an existence. It was at this point I gave Bridget the preview of her new and improved life. Bridget had nothing to lose except the weight she had gained and the prescription drugs she had been taking. She was ready to write her new life script.

"Not only did my test results indicate I was in early menopause (that had been masked by my birth control pill), but my other hormones were also messed up. I had vitamin deficiencies, thyroid issues and a litany of other problems that I can't even remember—there were that many of them. I remember sitting there thinking 'Oh my God!'

It took about one year to get me straightened out. Dr. Edwards took me off the birth control pills and gradually weaned me off the antidepressants.

Slowly, the depression started to lift and my blood pressure control improved. Getting off the anti-depressants was challenging, but Dr. Edwards put me on L-Theanine, and my whole mental picture improved. Logic finally returned to my thinking. When put into a bad or stressful situation, I could now think my way through it without flying off the handle and doing something irrational.

Bridget no longer required her anti-depressant or her blood pressure medication once her birth control pills were discontinued. The Theanine, coupled with exercise and yoga (see Chapter Nine), worked very well to keep her calm and alert. Once we corrected Bridget's hormonal imbalances, we found she had some other underlying issues:

"I discovered I had food allergies—something I had never been tested for. I had a gluten intolerance, which was inflaming my intestines and causing my body not to be able to absorb nutrients. Once I eliminated all of those foods from my diet, my IBS went away completely and I started losing weight. The bloating in my stomach and the aching in my joints went away, too. I am starting to get my sex drive back and I am not nearly as emotional as I used to be. I'm actually optimistic about my future rather than dreading getting out of bed every morning. For the areas of my life that need changing, I'm taking positive, logical steps to fix them rather than irrational, ineffective steps designed to "fill a hole" that never should have been there in the first place."

Bridget is more balanced, less medicated, less stressed, and now flourishing. She has written another book and is considering a career change since she has also realized the stress of being an attorney is a constant aggressor on her health. Bridget has lost weight, and her drive both sexually and professionally has returned.

BECOME THE VIP AT YOUR BODY'S HORMONE PARTY

By appreciating the synergy between your hormones and grasping their intricate connections and relationships, you are now better able to decipher your body's make-up and channel your stressors in a positive

LENA D. EDWARDS MD, FAARM

and productive direction. In other words, in order to preserve your mental and physical health, I suggest you become the VIP at your own party and assign your own "body guards" in the form of healthy living habits and stress-reducing life choices to ensure that your important party guests (your hormones) are respectful and civil to one another – and more importantly, to you!

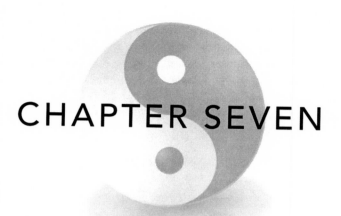

CHAPTER SEVEN

Too Much Of A Good Thing:
The Link Between High Cortisol and Disease

Stress is not what happens to us. It's our response TO what happens. And RESPONSE is something we can choose.

Maureen Killoran

Having read this far into Adrenalogic, you surely now appreciate how your stress levels can affect your sense of well-being, your ability to thrive, and your capacity to deal with the physical and emotional extremes your life offers. When you sleep well, eat well, engage in regular exercise, socialize with friends and family, and focus on the "positives" in life, you will be way ahead of those who don't.

Ultimately, our stress levels and how we perceive and react to stress are vitally important in determining whether we will remain healthy or become ill - <u>in more ways than most people realize</u>.

This chapter and the one following explain in detail how variations in the body's normal cortisol release patterns, extremes in cortisol output, and cortisol's effects on other hormones can not only cause annoying

LENA D. EDWARDS MD, FAARM

symptoms but also contribute to major medical issues such as autoimmune disease, cardiovascular disease, and diabetes. An understanding of the relationships between chronic stress and disease is imperative not only for patients but for physicians as well since approximately **75 - 90 percent of visits to primary care physicians are for stress-related problems.** By equipping yourself with this information, you can gain significant ground as you visit with your healthcare provider since time constraints now imposed on them have allowed for less time to delve into these issues with you.

In truth, patients' own time constraints also prevent them from adequately addressing and reducing stressors in their lives. Furthermore, the way in which we perceive stress puts us at risk of developing unhealthy 'coping' behaviours, such as smoking, over-eating, and excessive alcohol consumption. This only adds fuel to our stress-induced fire and further harms our bodies. So, next time you're poised to grab a hamburger and fries at the drive-thru because you're late getting home from the office, you might want to think about breaking this unhealthy chain of events now that you are more knowledgeable about the health effects of these behaviors.

UNCOVERING THE LINKS BETWEEN STRESS AND DISEASE

A comprehensive review of the medical literature reveals thousands of entries confirming an <u>evidence-based link between stress and the development of disease</u>. The *Journal of the American College of Cardiology*, April, 2008, stated, "There are extensive data concerning stressors' contributions to diverse pathophysiological changes including sudden death, myocardial infarction and ischemia (heart attacks and angina), heart motion abnormalities as well as to alterations in cardiac regulation."

Indeed, if you perform a quick web search using the key words "stress AND disease" you will find hundreds of pages of newspaper articles and university and medical studies all supporting a growing link between chronic stress and a multitude of diseases. Here are just a few examples:

- In a review of the scientific literature on the relationship between stress and disease, Carnegie Mellon University psychologist Sheldon Cohen has found that **stress is a contributing factor in human disease**, and in particular depression, cardiovascular disease and HIV/AIDS. (Psychological Stress and Disease, JAMA, 2007)
- A literature review published in the August 2007 issue of the *Journal of Periodontology* (JOP) saw a strong relationship between stress and periodontal diseases; 57 percent of the studies included in the review showed a positive relationship between periodontal diseases and psychological factors such as stress, distress, anxiety, depression, and loneliness. (ScienceDaily.com, 2007)
- Depression has many possible causes, likely related to genetics, brain chemicals and your life situation. Chronic stressful life situations can increase the risk of developing depression if you aren't coping with the stress well.

As we delve deeper into this topic, you will learn more about the physiologic effects of stress and abnormal cortisol production and the associations with many diseases including high blood pressure, peptic ulcer disease, migraine headaches, irritable bowel syndrome, impaired thyroid function, impaired immunity, memory loss, reproductive disorders, osteoporosis, mood disorders, diabetes, and premature aging.

HYPERCORTISOLISM: DISEASES AND DISORDERS RELATED TO HIGH CORTISOL

As we have discussed, cortisol production and release is under tight control or "regulation." **During times of acute stress, we need cortisol to divert the body's resources towards immediate survival and away from non-essential functions** such as feeding, sleeping, and reproducing. However, when elevated cortisol levels remain constant and the normal pattern of cortisol release disappears, hypercortisolism results. Think about it this way: You're writing a critical final exam in order to graduate from your university – every day for four months! This highly stressful situation means that your body can't keep up with the continual call for it to be on "high alert."

There are numerous ways through which a chronically-elevated cortisol state can arise such as the exam scenario mentioned above. Suffice it to say that the normal mechanisms of allostasis (the process of adapting through change to regain balance, as discussed in Chapter One) can go awry. The result? A locomotive train in motion with no brakes. Those near the train tracks: Beware!

Here are the ways in which some key body systems react to stress:

1 NERVOUS SYSTEM

When stressed - physically or psychologically - the body suddenly shifts its energy resources to fighting off the perceived threat. In what is known as the "fight or flight" response, the sympathetic nervous system signals the adrenal glands to release adrenaline and cortisol. These hormones make the heart beat faster. raise blood pressure, change the digestive process and boost glucose levels in the bloodstream. Once the crisis passes, body systems usually return to normal.

2 MUSCULOSKELETAL SYSTEM

Under stress, muscles tense up. The contraction of muscles for extended periods can trigger tension headaches, migraines and various musculoskeletal conditions.

3 RESPIRATORY SYSTEM

Stress can make you breathe harder and cause rapid breathing - or hyperventilation - which can bring on panic attacks in some people.

4 CARDIOVASCULAR SYSTEM

Acute stress - stress that is momentary, such as being stuck in traffic -

causes an increase in heart rate and stronger contractions of the heart muscle. Blood vessels that direct blood to the large muscles and to the heart dilate, increasing the amount of blood pumped to these parts of the body. Repeated episodes of acute stress can cause inflammation in the coronary arteries, thought to lead to heart attack.

⑤ ENDOCRINE SYSTEM

Adrenal Glands - When the body is stressed, the brain sends signals from the hypothalamus, causing the adrenal cortex to produce cortisol and the adrenal medulla to produce epinephrine - sometimes called the "stress hormones."

Liver - When cortisol and epinephrine are released, the liver produces more glucose, a blood sugar that would give you the energy for "fight or flight" in an emergency.

⑥ GASTROINTESTINAL SYSTEM

Esophagus - Stress may prompt you to eat much more or much less than you usually do. If you eat more of different foods or increase your use of tobacco or alcohol, you may experience heartburn, or acid reflux.

Stomach - Your stomach can react with "butterflies" or even nausea or pain. You may vomit if the stress is severe enough.

Bowels - Stress can affect digestion and which nutrients your intestines absorb. It can also affect how quickly food moves through your body. You may find that you have either diarrhea or constipation.

⑦ REPRODUCTIVE SYSTEM

In men, excess amounts of cortisol, produced under stress, can affect the normal functioning of the reproductive system. Chronic stress can impair testosterone and sperm production and cause impotence.

In women, stress can cause absent or irregular menstrual cycles or more-painful periods. It can also reduce sexual desire.

The graphic and information above from The Washington Post

If you recall our discussion of "hormone synergy" from Chapter Six, you probably aren't surprised by any of the consequences of excess

LENA D. EDWARDS MD, FAARM

cortisol states. A quick review will remind you of some of these hormone interrelationships (or those dysfunctional party minglers) and how they are partially responsible for some of the metabolic and clinical consequences of hypercortisolism. These include:

- Inhibition of **growth hormone** production (i.e. the onset of osteoporosis, decreased muscle mass, decreased sense of well-being, obesity)
- Interference with **thyroid hormone** action (i.e. experiencing fatigue, constipation, high cholesterol, high blood pressure)
- Interference with **insulin action** (i.e. weight gain, the development of metabolic syndrome, diabetes)
- Interference with **reproductive hormone production** and function (i.e. irregular or absent menstruation, infertility, impotence)

I remind you of these associations so that you better understand how and why stress causes *such a diverse array of symptoms*. So, as one example, even if you are convinced your fatigue and hair loss are caused by malfunction of your thyroid gland but your lab results are "within range," remember that high cortisol can lower thyroid hormone *production and conversion*. Through this understanding, it may then seem plausible that correcting your hypercortisolism is essential to correcting your "functional hypothyroidism" (see Glossary).

The table below highlights some common conditions which have been associated with increased HPA axis activity and hypercortisolism:

CHRONIC STRESS	ALCOHOL WITHDRAWAL
MAJOR DEPRESSION	NARCOTIC WITHDRAWAL
ANOREXIA NERVOSA	FUNCTIONAL BOWEL DISEASE
MALNUTRITION	OBESITY
OBSESSIVE-COMPULSIVE DISORDER	METABOLIC SYNDROME X
PANIC DISORDER	CHILDHOOD SEXUAL STATURE
EXCESSIVE EXERCISE	PSYCHOSOCIAL SHORT STATURE
CHRONIC ACTIVE ALCOHOLISM	HYPERTHYROIDISM

Reference for table: Chrousos & Gold. JAMA. 1992; 267: 1244-125

Intriguing, isn't it: The incredible connections between our organs, chronic stress, increased HPA axis activity, and high cortisol? Well, what you have read thus far is just the tip of the "stress iceberg." It gets even more interesting...

HEART DISEASE

The process through which hypercortisolism promotes heart disease is complex and multi-dimensional. However, **several studies have linked <u>emotional stress</u> to sudden cardiac death in 20 to 40 percent of patients!** The recipe for potential cardiac "disaster" calls for several ingredients, all of which are either directly or indirectly influenced by the actions of cortisol.

- A key ingredient is **cortisol-induced growth hormone deficiency**. Since growth hormone is essential in maintaining heart health, a deficiency in this hormone has been shown to impair heart structure and function, increase cholesterol, and increase inflammation.
- Another essential component is **high blood sugar**. Recall that cortisol is the primary hormone that controls your carbohydrate metabolism. It is responsible for pulling out all the stops when it comes to fueling your escape.
- Add to the above ingredients: **inflammation, high blood pressure, high cholesterol, blood vessel 'dysfunction', and susceptibility to blood clotting** ('thrombus' formation) within the arteries and you end up with a 'perfect storm' if you will.

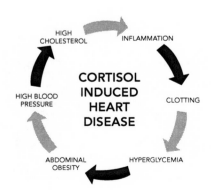

LENA D. EDWARDS MD, FAARM

We discussed **work stress** in Chapter Three, but could too much work or too much stress on the job actually damage our hearts? The answer is yes. One landmark study showing such an association between work, stress, and health was conducted in England in 2002. *The Whitehall II Study* included 10,000 male and female participants aged thirty-five to fifty-five who worked as civil servants in twenty government departments. During the five years the study subjects were followed, **researchers found a definite association between heart disease and chronic work-related stress**. They also reported that stressed workers were more prone to poor diet, higher cortisol levels, physical inactivity, and metabolic syndrome. Their conclusion was that "work stress may be an important determinant of coronary heart disease." So, again, if your work days consist of constant deadlines, overtime, skipping meals or indulging in unhealthy vending machine snacks – you may be playing a serious game of Russian Roulette with your heart.

Other job-related factors associated with future or even premature heart disease include lack of control over one's job, job strain, high job demands, and lack of autonomy. To add insult to injury, chronic stress (in the form of fatigue, irritability, and demoralization) and hostility have been tied to activation of the clotting system which also has been shown to increase the risk of heart attack. In addition, feelings of exhaustion and emotional stress can contribute to the development of high blood pressure via activation of the HPA axis. There's an interesting tie-in here for you philosophy buffs... Remember Karl Marx's idea about workers provided with menial or trivial tasks in the workplace? They have little control over the final "product," and this can result in alienation. We can see how little this concept has changed over time!

ALZHEIMER'S DISEASE

We have not spent much time discussing cortisol's effects on the brain, but I can sum it up in one word... **frightening**! Many different areas of the brain are affected by cortisol, but one area in particular, the hippocampus, has very high levels of cortisol receptors and therefore is damaged under the influence of chronically high levels of cortisol. If you value your memory, the hippocampus is one brain structure you do not want to be without. The hippocampus also serves a very important role in regulating the stress response system and inhibiting the HPA axis and cortisol release.

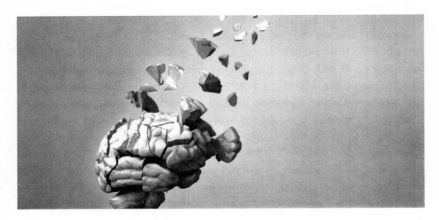

In Alzheimer's disease, a neurodegenerative disease that affects almost five million people in the U.S. alone, the hippocampus is one of the first regions of the brain to suffer damage. Impaired memory and disorientation are among the first symptoms to appear. There is growing evidence that the effects of physical and psychosocial stressors on the HPA axis may be implicated in the onset and progression of Alzheimer's disease.

MOOD DISORDERS

Feeling down? You're not alone. According to the *National Institute of Mental Health*, Approximately 20.9 million American adults, or about 9.5 percent of the U.S. population age eighteen and older (median age is thirty), are diagnosed with a mood disorder in a given year. Sadly, mental disorders are the leading cause of disability in the U.S. and Canada. According to a government study done by the Center for Disease Control, anti-depressants have become the most commonly prescribed drugs in the United States. In fact, anti-depressants are prescribed more often than drugs to treat high blood pressure, high cholesterol, asthma, or headaches <u>combined</u>.

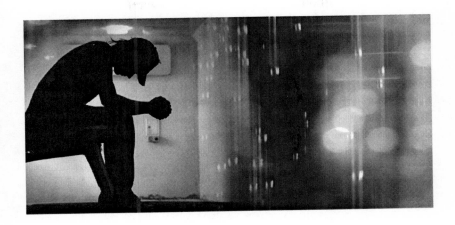

Among all psychiatric disorders, generalized anxiety and depression are the two that are most often stress-related. Although other stress hormones also play a role, cortisol is the primary instigator in this regard. It is believed that the "cortisol conundrum" that occurs in mood disorders arises not only because the cortisol's "on/off" switch does not get turned off but also because the cortisol receptors in your brain are not properly functioning.

Furthermore, an extensive review of the medical literature also reveals an association between a hyperactive HPA axis (high cortisol) and these other mood disorders:

- Borderline personality disorder
- ADHD or attention-deficit/hyperactivity disorder
- Schizophrenia
- Depression
- Bipolar disorder
- Drug addiction
- Anxiety
- Autism

If you have ever complained of depression or anxiety to your doctor, you may have been prescribed a SSRI drug (selective serotonin reuptake inhibitor) like Prozac, Celexa, Zoloft, and Lexapro. These drugs *do not directly raise serotonin levels.* Rather, they basically work to keep the serotonin your nerve cells are already making hang around longer by preventing its "re-uptake," hence their name. In actuality, it is believed these drugs probably help mood disorders by affecting *cortisol levels* more so than the levels of serotonin and other brain chemicals. SSRIs restore the function of cortisol's receptors and turn off the "on" switch. The overall effect is to lower levels of cortisol which then improves the depression. Research in this area is ongoing, and on the horizon are anti-depressant drugs capable of indirectly lowering cortisol's tissue effects by improving cortisol *receptor* function.

OSTEOPOROSIS

Osteoporosis, a condition which results in thinning of bone tissue and reduced bone density, affects an estimated 75 million people in Europe, USA and Japan. By the year 2050, the worldwide incidence of hip fracture is projected to increase by 310 percent in men and 240 percent in women. In white women, the lifetime risk of hip fracture is one in six, compared with a one in nine risk of a diagnosis of breast cancer. Clearly, research on the available drugs has shown a favourable outcome in treating osteoporosis, but isn't being proactive a more rational and cost-effective approach?

As you have already learned, excess cortisol is to bone what kryptonite is to Superman – a powerful deterrent to growth and strength. In fact, in patients who have Cushing's Disease, researchers have found that hypercortisolism may cause spinal fractures in up to 70 percent of patients. Excess cortisol:

- Inhibits bone formation
- Prevents your gut from absorbing calcium
- Increases bone breakdown
- Lowers the levels of hormones and other growth factors that help to build bone

In osteoporosis patients who *do not* have Cushing's Disease, subtle hypercortisolism is more common than most healthcare professionals recognize. In fact, studies have shown that **up to 10 percent of the general population manifest osteoporosis as their only symptom of otherwise silent hypercortisolism**. As such, the diagnosis of hypercortisolism must be ruled out in patients who have unexplained osteoporosis.

DIABETES AND METABOLIC SYNDROME

Years of scientific research suggest that patients with metabolic syndrome and diabetes have high HPA axis activity/hypercortisolism and that **stress may play an important role**. More than four hundred years ago, the famous English physician Thomas Willis noted that diabetes often occurred in patients who had experienced significant life stresses, sadness, or long standing sorrow. **More recent research has shown there to be a link between the development of diabetes and work stress, distressed sleep, anger/hostility, traumatic events, and general emotional stress.**

Stress contributes to the development of abnormal blood sugar regulation in several ways, some of which include:

- Behavioral mechanisms
- Smoking
- Excessive and unhealthy eating
- Lack of exercise
- Alcohol abuse
- Physiological insulin resistance
- Increased HPA axis activity
- Increased SNS activity (catecholamines)
- Increased abdominal fat accumulation
- Increased levels of inflammation

You will recall that cortisol is the hormone that directly and indirectly raises blood sugar. So, if your cortisol is chronically elevated, so too will your glucose be.

Metabolic syndrome, a precursor to diabetes, is a grouping of medical conditions in which a patient has at least three of the following common abnormalities:

- Central obesity (fat deposition in the mid section)
- High blood pressure
- Insulin resistance
- Low HDL (good) cholesterol

- High triglycerides

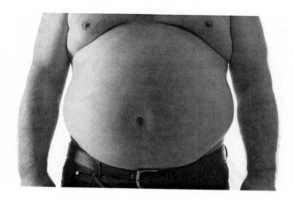

Not only does metabolic syndrome or "MeS" predispose a person to becoming diabetic, it is also associated with an increased risk of heart disease and premature death. One-fourth of the world's adult population now has metabolic syndrome! And...

- People with MeS are **twice** as likely to die from a stroke or heart attack and **five times more likely** to develop Type 2 diabetes.
- Of the approximate 285 million people around the world with diabetes, **80 percent** will die from heart disease.
- MeS and diabetes cause more disease and death than HIV/AIDS. (International Diabetes Federation)

Since stress raises blood sugar and blocks the body from releasing insulin in people with Type 2 diabetes, stress reduction and lifestyle modification are particularly important in these patients. Moreover, patients with diabetes are even more susceptible to the harmful effects of cortisol than are non-diabetics.

Now might be a good time to tell you Jason's story so we can reinforce what you have learned so far. Jason, a fifty-nine-year-old business executive, is the perfect example of someone who was heading towards certain cortisol-induced annihilation. Here's Jason's story, told from his perspective... perhaps YOU can relate.

LENA D. EDWARDS MD. FAARM

WHEN CORTISOL TAKES OVER:
JASON'S STORY

"I was always ahead of my game, always at the top. I started my own company when I was only twenty-five and built it into a huge business. At first, I loved the challenges, the opportunities, and the end results. Unfortunately, the business eventually turned into a monster which began slowly consuming me about ten years ago.

The changes were subtle at first. Fit turned to flab as exercise became another entry on my "to-do" list. My mental stealth was dwindling into mental mush as I struggled to remember times, dates, and names.

My fuse had become extremely short, and I would yell at people left and right for minor mistakes. My wife became increasingly irritated with me. The fact that my sex drive had taken a nose dive made this latter problem less of an issue. But thanks to my insomnia, all the nights I spent on the couch were not wasted: I was able to get work done, watch old movies, and count the ceiling tiles in the family room.

I took great pride in my success. I owned a company with several subsidiaries and over two hundred employees. I used to thrive on that kind of stress. But over time, I hit the wall... Maybe it was my age or maybe it was the fact that the stress in my personal life had escalated to very high levels. One day a long time and very astute friend of mine took me to lunch. He was brutally honest with me, but I now thank him for saving my life. He said that through working with a new doctor, he was able to remedy many of his problems and was even able to identify potential problems and head them off before they became major health concerns. He told me that although the process would be gradual, it would be well worth the wait. At the age of sixty-two, he was feeling better "than he ever had in his life!"

So, I sucked it up and went to see his doctor, Dr. Edwards. After a fairly extensive discussion with her, she initially recommended blood work, a urine collection, and a saliva test to check hormones and other basics as a first step. She told me that while we were waiting for results, I could try taking a supplement called inositol (see Glossary) to help with anxiety and sleep. If that didn't work, she suggested I try something called 5-HTP (see Chapter Nine).

She briefly explained some of the consequences of chronic stress and high cortisol levels and she was able to provide me with legitimate medical explanations for how this one pervasive problem and its wide spread effects could be fueling many of my symptoms. She also gave me a few articles on stress, cortisol, and health to review in the meantime.

When I saw Dr. Edwards to review my test results, my anxiety was actually better. The 5-HTP I was taking allowed me a straight four hours of sleep! Not surprisingly, my saliva and twenty-four hour urine collection showed that my cortisol levels were very high. Dr. Edwards explained how this alone could contribute to my high blood pressure, insomnia, anxiety, muscle loss, and belly fat. The rest of my results were not pretty either. My blood sugar was too high, I had a lot of low vitamin levels, my testosterone was too low, my estrogen was too high and my DHEA was low. I also now had high cholesterol which I had never had a problem with before.

To prevent me from spontaneously combusting, Dr. Edwards recommended I take some time off work. Although I was convinced my business could not run without me, magically it did. Over the next three months, her treatment plan included:

- Low impact exercises (yoga and Pilates) with some weight training,
- A radical change in my diet (good-bye to alcohol, refined sugar, and fried foods), sleep hygiene (regular sleep/wake times), and meditation.
- She also used the supplements phosphatidylserine and ashwaganda to help control my cortisol levels. I was also put on vitamins, omega 3 fatty acids, and a probiotic. She also started me on a topical bio-equivalent hormone cream which contained testosterone and DHEA. Dr. Edwards told me that adding these hormones would optimize my deficient levels as well as lower my cortisol levels.

The first three months were tough, especially trying to comply with strict go to sleep and wake up times. Luckily a sleep study did not show any sleep apnea or restless leg syndrome. But in just that short period of time,

LENA D. EDWARDS MD, FAARM

I felt 75 percent better. Dr. Edwards allowed me to return to a part-time work schedule after the first three weeks but gave me strict guidelines about the number of hours and levels of stress to which I could be exposed. She told me that I would never get better and/or I would definitely suffer from a relapse if I returned to my previous high stress, fast-paced work schedule. One year later, I find myself in the same position as the friend who sent me to see Dr. Edwards. I feel better than I have in years. I gained insight into how my life was killing me and have tried not to go back there. Sure, I fall off the wagon and eat junk food on occasion or have a few glasses of wine with dinner, but I am careful not to let it get out of hand. And I have since hired a CEO for my business so that I still have an income but, more importantly, I have more time with my family and more peace of mind. And, thanks to Dr. Edwards, I now have my health back."

IMMUNE SYSTEM

Your immune system is designed to protect you from foreign invaders, be they food particles, viruses, bacteria, or cancer cells. **Cortisol has an enormous influence over immune system function and vice versa**. When your immune system is stimulated, the HPA axis gets the "green light" and up goes cortisol. You might be surprised to know that the reason cortisol goes up is to protect your immune system from doing too good a job and destroying your own healthy tissue along with the intruders.

There are many different cell types called into active duty when your immune response is put on high alert. When cortisol comes along, it breaks up the action by reducing the activity, population, production, and activation of immune system cells. Now, this is a great thing in the short term. Self-destruction is a bad thing. But what happens when cortisol doesn't take its foot off the brake?

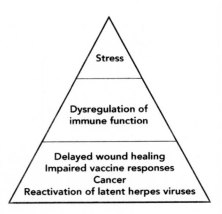

Data from: Webster, Marketon JI and Glaser, R. Stress Hormones and Immune Function. Cell Immunol. 2008 Mar-Apr 252 (1-2): 16-26 Epub 2008.)

Notice the word *cancer* in the above pyramid. Yes... **Stress has been shown to influence the incidence and progression of cancer**. In fact, epidemiological and clinical studies over the past thirty years have provided strong evidence for links between chronic stress, depression and social isolation, and cancer progression. Chronic stress not only prevents proper function of the immune cells that kill cancer cells, it has also been shown to prevent your DNA from repairing itself when it becomes damaged.

Behavioral oncologists (see Glossary) have described a "Type C" personality which encompasses such behaviours as denial and suppression of emotions, particularly anger. Other personality characteristics of Type C 'cancer prone' individuals are:

- Avoidance of conflicts
- Exaggerated social desirability
- Harmonizing behaviour (forcing oneself to fit in with others)
- Over-compliance
- Over-patience
- High rationality
- Rigid control of emotional expression

These behavioural patterns usually appear to be effective as long as

LENA D. EDWARDS MD, FAARM

environmental and psychological balance is maintained. But, this delicate balance is easily disrupted under the impact of accumulated stressors, especially those that make people feel depressed, helpless, or hopeless. This is the perfect way to demonstrate the point made earlier about how it is not simply the stressor **but your reaction to the stressor** that dictates whether or not you're your stress will ultimately harm you. It's hard to believe that by simply reacting differently to tense or difficult situations may save your life. If you're the type of person who tends to fly off the handle easily, you may need to rethink your perspective. Conversely, if you're the type who avoids conflict at all costs, you may need to learn to speak up.

PREMATURE AGING

A hugely popular movement which seems to be skyrocketing is "anti-aging." It seems ironic that some people spend incredible amounts of money to remove, refill, inject, nip, and tuck their way back to youth. Although some may think aging is only skin deep, the truth of the matter is that what happens on the outside is merely a reflection of what is going on inside.

An entire book could be written on how stress and high cortisol contribute to premature aging both inside and out. Have you heard the term "free radicals" before? Free radicals are those nasty little molecules that wreak havoc inside your cells if not properly neutralized. The result (in medical jargon) is known as "oxidative stress." This is essentially internal rusting of your cells... *All of your cells.* Hence, we have all been forewarned and advised to consume more *anti-oxidants* or "rust retardants" to neutralize free radicals thus preventing aging and disease.

The process of internal and external rusting is fueled by, you guessed it, cortisol. Growing numbers of studies reveal that markers of oxidative stress (or internal rusting) are increased by both acute and chronic stress, particularly stress that is psychological in nature. So, to summarize:

high cortisol + oxidative stress (DNA and cell damage) + inflammation + low anabolic hormone levels = *premature aging*

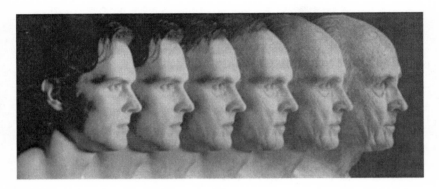

Where are you in the aging continuum?

OBESITY

We've mentioned unhealthy eating habits quite a few times in *Adrenalogic*, and it's for a good reason. Obesity - something the World Health Organization (WHO) defines as "abnormal or excessive fat accumulation that may impair health" is a growing epidemic.

The term *body mass index*, or BMI, may be familiar to you as a measurement of obesity. BMI is a simple index of weight-for-height that is commonly used in classifying overweight and obesity in adults and is defined as the weight in kilograms divided by the square of the height in meters (kg/m^2). A person is considered obese if their BMI is greater than thirty.

You may want to sit down (or better yet: stand up and do some yoga stretches!) before you peruse these numbers. The latest projections from the WHO indicate that globally in 2005:

- Approximately 1.6 billion adults (age 15+) were overweight
- At least 400 million adults were obese
- By 2015, approximately 2.3 billion adults will be overweight and more than 700 million will be obese
- At least 20 million children under the age of 5 years were overweight

LENA D. EDWARDS MD. FAARM

- The incidence of obesity in the U.S. has doubled in the last decade

These statistics are *very bad news*, unless of course you earn your living selling bariatric (weight loss) surgical devices or obesity drugs, the sales of which have quadrupled in the past five years alone!

Let's talk about what simple high cortisol does to your body in terms of fat accumulation and distribution.

Abdominal fat is a fantastic target tissue for stress. Stress, particularly psychological stress, has been related to obesity in numerous studies. Depending on your waist circumference and your levels of stress, you may have already discovered that cortisol makes fat cells in the abdomen grow and multiply. Mounting evidence suggests that:

- Abdominal fat deposition is related to greater psychological vulnerability to stress and impaired coping
- Stress-induced cortisol secretion may contribute to belly fat and all of the health consequences thereof

HIGH CORTISOL + HIGH INSULIN =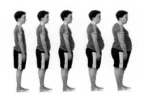

Also keep in mind that insulin is a co-conspirator in this assault. Cortisol raises the levels of insulin, and when these two hormones are present in high amounts, your belly fat cells are essentially doomed. Bottom line: Stress can make you fat and being fat can make you stressed.

SLEEP DISTURBANCES

Perhaps the best example of a "vicious circle" is that between stress and sleep disturbances. Stress, along with depression, anxiety, and tension are among the most common causes of sleep deprivation. A chronic sleep-restricted state can cause not only annoying symptoms, like fatigue, foggy thinking, and clumsiness; it can lead to even more detrimental consequences such as diabetes and obesity.

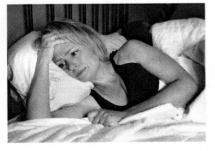

According to the Better Sleep Council, 65 percent of Americans are losing sleep secondary to stress. Current events, personal finances, and family issues account for nearly half of stress induced sleep losses.

Chronic sleep deprivation, whether in the form of insomnia, sleep apnea, or other sleep disturbance, can result in any of the following:

EFFECTS OF SLEEP DEPRIVATION

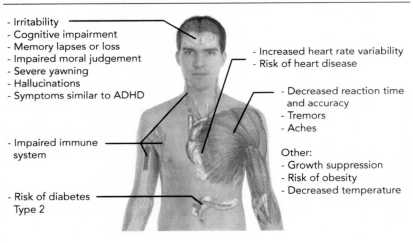

- Irritability
- Cognitive impairment
- Memory lapses or loss
- Impaired moral judgement
- Severe yawning
- Hallucinations
- Symptoms similar to ADHD

- Increased heart rate variability
- Risk of heart disease

- Decreased reaction time and accuracy
- Tremors
- Aches

- Impaired immune system

Other:
- Growth suppression
- Risk of obesity
- Decreased temperature

- Risk of diabetes Type 2

Information in graphic from Morin, Charles M. (2003) Insomnia. New York: Kluwer Academic Publ. p. 28, National Institutes of Neurologic Disease and Stroke and Wikipedia

People with sleep disturbances have been found to have abnormal elevations in their night time cortisol levels. In fact, you may notice that the list of symptoms of sleep deprivation is almost identical to those of hypercortisolism. Furthermore, many of the daytime symptoms caused by sleep disturbances are also fueled by increased levels of inflammation.

LENA D. EDWARDS MD. FAARM

Remember the cortisol/immune system connection?

Breaking this cycle involves identifying the cause of the sleep disturbance, maintaining normal sleep/wake cycles, and reducing or eliminating the stressors keeping you awake. We will discuss this in more detail when we discuss ways to "outsmart" stress in Chapter Nine.

It's scary, isn't it: To think that chronic stress has the potential to wreak so much havoc on our bodies, our health, our relationships, our lives? But, the good news is that we do have some control over its impact; we can choose how to respond to situations, we can make health conscious choices (including reading books like this), and we can set an example and teach our children how to manage their health now and in the future. Towards the end of the book, I reveal more detailed advice and tips on how to best counter HPA axis dysfunction, stress, and stress-related disease through lifestyle, diet, spiritual, health and relationship opportunities.

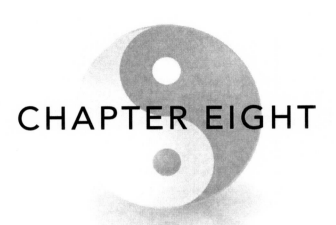

CHAPTER EIGHT

Not Enough Of A Good Thing: The Link Between Low Cortisol And Disease

"You don't know what you've got till it's gone"
Cinderella (Rock Group)

While you may still be in awe at the destructive power of chronic cortisol excess, try to now imagine the opposite situation... what would happen if your daytime cortisol was *chronically low*?

When we take a closer look at a host of common stress-related diseases and disorders, we find that low cortisol frequently comes into play. In fact, **hypocortisolism (defined below) has been found in 20 to 25 percent of patient with these stress-related bodily disorders:**

- Chronic fatigue syndrome
- Fibromyalgia
- Irritable bowel syndrome
- PTSD
- Burnout
- Chronic pain

LENA D. EDWARDS MD, FAARM

- Atypical depression

Interestingly, there appears to be very specific groups of patients in whom low-cortisol levels in the morning and abnormally low cortisol release during the day are more often seen. They include:

- Teachers living under chronic stress suffering from burnout
- White collar workers with high degrees of job stress
- Mothers of toddlers who have insecure attachments
- Those who work excessive numbers of hours outside the home
- Children who have experienced trauma or are in neglectful environments

So exactly what is **Hypocortisolism**? It can be defined as:

1.) An abnormally low or flat daytime cortisol pattern; and/or

2.) A condition in which your body fails to produce an appropriate rise in cortisol in response to a stressor

And exactly how does this situation arise? Is it because your adrenal glands just decide to hang it up and quit working? No! There are actually a number of theories on how chronically low cortisol states develop. Chapter Four provided you with a preview of a few pathways leading to low cortisol, and I am going to elaborate on this a bit more so as to further drive home one of the book's main points... *Primary adrenal failure due to chronic stress has not been scientifically proven.* Rather, it is primarily via dysfunction or under activity of the HPA axis that hypocortisolism is born. However, other mechanisms have also been demonstrated as we will discuss below.

One theory: hypocortisolism ultimately occurs after an initial phase of constant hyperactivity of the HPA axis. In this scenario, your stress response system resembles a car... It can only be driven for so long and so fast before it will eventually run out of gas.

In other situations, hypocortisolism becomes the body's "new norm" as an adaptive response to chronic stress. It has been shown that exposure to a psycho-social stressor over and over again often results in a decrease in cortisol response. Your body's stress speakers essentially dial the volume down to prevent excessive noise.

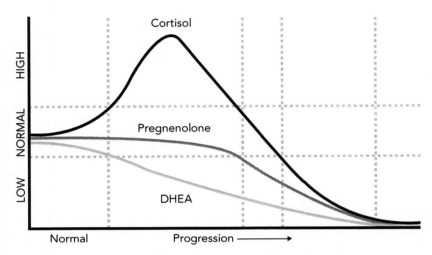

TIME OF EACH STAGE IS HIGHLY VARIABLE

Below are some illustrations of what years of research have shown to be potential causes of hypocortisolism. The following is the abbreviated version:

1. **Centrally mediated** (Causes that stem from within the brain)

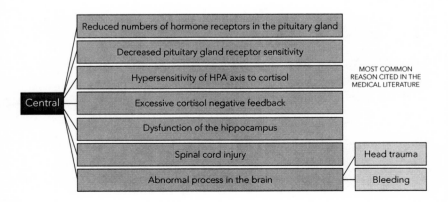

LENA D. EDWARDS MD, FAARM

2. **Peripherally mediated** (Causes that stem from areas below the brain)

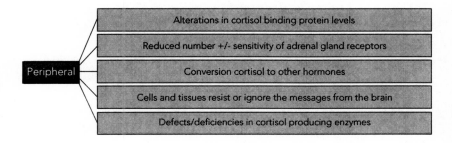

3. **Adrenally mediated** (Causes that stem from the adrenal glands)

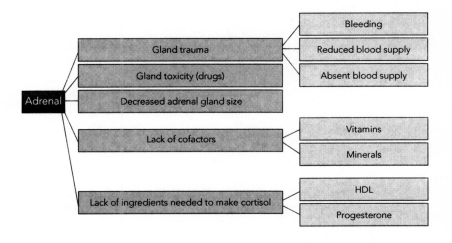

PROTECTIVE MEASURES?

Although perhaps difficult to conceive, **the state of low cortisol may actually be beneficial**. Consider what happens when you are under attack by a virus or bacteria. Cortisol goes up to make sure your overly anxious immune system doesn't destroy your own healthy cells (recall this discussion from Chapter Seven). In the face of an infection, you might consider suppressing the immune system to be counter intuitive, especially in a situation when the immune attack is prolonged or repetitive. So what would a reduction in cortisol accomplish? Essentially, it would remove the cortisol "blockade" thereby allowing your immune defenses to overthrow the attempted viral or bacterial coup d'état. You see, a <u>healthy immune system in full force is no match against any invader</u>.

Remember how horrible you feel when you are sick? Have you ever had the pleasure of experiencing the flu? Now consider the concept of the "sickness response," a term described by Dr. Hart in the late 1980's to describe non-specific symptoms such as fatigue, increased sensitivity to pain, difficulty concentrating, depressed mood, and decreased appetite often seen during an infection. So what if your body was actually making you feel miserable *to save you*? Some believe that the sickness response may actually represent an adaptive "reorganization" of priorities if you will: conserve energy, destroy the infection, and survive first... Eat, think, and be merry later. Our body's ability to adapt is far-reaching and amazingly complex.

Finally, other known causes of low hypocortisolism include liver disease (cirrhosis) and critical illness. In some people, low cortisol can even be a normal variant, causing no trouble or symptoms whatsoever. Again, I propose to you: How do you feel about the term "adrenal fatigue" now?

SYMPTOMS OF HYPOCORTISOLISM

The three most common symptoms (the "symptom triad" if you will) seen in patients with hypocortisolism are: **sensitivity to stress, pain, and chronic fatigue.** However, other signs and symptoms can also be seen which resemble those of Addison's Disease even though they are not as severe. It is for this reason that some in the medical community have nicknamed hypocortisolism "subclinical Addison's Disease."

The table below summarizes some of the major symptoms seen in patients with low cortisol states.

TABLE 1: SIGNS AND SYMPTOMS OF HYPOCORTISOLISM
General: fatigue, fever, weakness, muscle pain, joint pain, sore throat, headaches, dizziness upon standing, chronic pain
Gastrointestinal: Lack of appetite, nausea, vomiting, diarrhea, abdominal or flank pain
Psychiatric: Depression, apathy, irritability, sleep disturbances, difficulty concentrating, difficulty with memory, confusion, stress sensitivity
Cardiovascular: Increased heart rate, abnormal regulation of blood pressure and heart rate with changes in body position, dehydration, depressed heart contractions
Laboratory: Low blood sugar, low sodium, high potassium, high calcium, increased numbers of white blood cells, elevated prolactin levels, hypothyroidism

Because many of these same signs and symptoms are seen in other medical conditions, patients with hypocortisolism often go undiagnosed or are simply diagnosed with chronic fatigue syndrome or depression. It is in these situations that the astute healthcare professional expands the differential diagnosis by assessing the functionality of the patient's HPA axis.

Here's an example of a Janice's salivary cortisol results (the patient discussed below). As you can see, her cortisol levels are consistently low throughout the day when compared to an individual with a healthy stress response system.

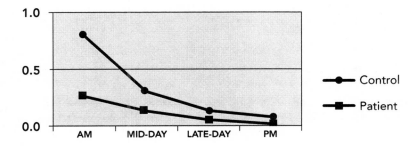

As with hypercortisolism, a bevy of modern-day diseases are linked to hypocortisolism. They include the following conditions:

ATYPICAL DEPRESSION	AFTER CHRONIC STRESS
CHRONIC FATIGUE SYNDROME	POSTPARTUM PERIOD
FIBROMYALGIA	RHEUMATOID ARTHRITIS
HYPOTHYROIDISM	MENOPAUSE
NICOTINE WITHDRAWAL	PMS/PMDD

Given everything we have already discussed, these disease associations should now make complete sense. I now want to provide you with more evidence-based research and insight about some of the very common conditions linked with low cortisol states.

CHRONIC FATIGUE SYNDROME

Chronic fatigue syndrome (CFS) is defined as clinically unexplained, persistent, or relapsing fatigue of at least six month's duration and the presence of at least four of these symptoms:

- Sore throat
- Tender, enlarged lymph nodes in neck or under arm region
- Muscle pain
- Pain in multiple joints
- Fatigue after exercise
- Non-refreshing sleep
- Headaches
- Impaired memory/concentration

Studies estimate that the prevalence of CFS in adults is between 0.5 and 5 percent with the majority of sufferers being women. Since there is currently no effective treatment for this debilitating condition, it's important for us to fully understand the underlying causes. **Some of us in the field of integrative medicine do not believe CFS is an independent disease** state but rather a clinical consequence of one or more lurking problems.

The culprits may include:

- Mitochondrial (sources of cellular energy) dysfunction
- Sleep disorders
- Immune system dysfunction
- Chronic infections
- Gastrointestinal dysfunction
- Abnormalities in the clotting system
- Autonomic nervous system malfunction

So where is the "disconnect" in CFS patients? Well, several mechanisms have been identified:

- Reduced baseline HPA axis function
- Decreased function or abnormal regulation of HPA axis
- Blunted (flattened) morning cortisol levels
- Inappropriately low stimulated cortisol levels
- Elevated levels of inflammation

A key point here is that the majority of the medical evidence does not find primary adrenal gland failure to be the cause of low cortisol in CFS patients. As an example, a 2008 issue of the *Journal of Chronic Fatigue Syndrome* published an evidence based review of CFS and fibromyalgia by Dr. Kent Holtorf. After his review of the medical literature, he notes:

"... A more important fact is, however, that a multitude of studies have demonstrated the HPA axis dysfunction in these conditions [CFS and fibromyalgia] is central (hypothalamic or pituitary), not a primary adrenal insufficiency."

Finally, I want to share with you the interesting observations of Dr. Ricardo Baschetti of Italy. Over the past decade, he has written extensively on the association between low cortisol states and CFS and has been quite vocal in his belief that CFS actually represents a form of subclinical Addison's Disease. He supports his views by highlighting the fact that in comparing CFS to Addison's Disease, there is an apparent overlap of forty-three clinical symptoms, a phenomenon that is clearly not coincidental. In a 2005 Letter to the Editor of the *Journal of Internal Medicine*, Dr. Baschetti writes:

"Considering that most features of CFS, such as debilitating fatigue, an abrupt onset precipitated by a stressor, feverishness, arthralgias, myalgias, adenopathy, postexertional fatigue, exacerbation of allergic responses, and disturbances in mood and sleep are all characteristic of glucocorticoid [cortisol] insufficiency, it is not surprising that hypocortisolism has been convincingly shown to be implicated in the pathophysiology of CFS."

FIBROMYALGIA

According to the National Fibromyalgia Association, fibromyalgia (FM) is one of the most common chronic pain conditions, affecting approximately 10 million people in the U.S. and an estimated 3 to 6 percent of the worldwide population. Although patients of all ages, genders, and ethnicities can be affected, 75 to 90 percent of them are women. The risk of acquiring FM increases with age so that by age eighty, approximately 8 percent of adults meet the American College of Rheumatology classification of fibromyalgia.

Similar to CFS, FM is characterized by:

- Widespread, chronic muscle pain
- Increased sensitivity to touch
- Fatigue
- Sleep disturbances
- Morning stiffness

FM sufferers also report more depression, anxiety, and psychosocial stress. FM often coexists with CFS, probably because the mechanisms through which both conditions arise are in parallel. However, FM patients also tend to be deficient not only in cortisol but also in androgens (testosterone and DHEA), thyroid hormone, growth hormone, and catecholamines.

To illustrate further, in 2003, Kivimaki and colleagues conducted a study of FM in 4791 hospital employees and found that work related stress (high workload, victimization of bullying, lack of control over decision making) seemed to be a contributing factor in the development of FM. However, in this and other studies, other important variables have been identified. They include:

LENA D. EDWARDS MD, FAARM

- **Psychological predisposition**
  - Emotional neglect
  - Victimization
  - Problems with school or vocation
- **Biological predisposition**
  - Genetic make up
  - Temperament
  - Early pain or disease experiences

These factors, coupled with family or job stress and a lack of ability to cope, essentially create the perfect fibromyalgia "storm."

Now would be a good time to share Janice's story with you (whose salivary cortisol graph is on page 117). Janice, like many other patients suffering from FM, endured her symptoms with quiet valour, attempting not to inconvenience her friends and family members. She had long ago lost hope that modern medicine would find a cure for her FM since so many of her test results and treatment trials had failed.

JANICE'S STORY

Janice was a young woman who came to see me because of unrelenting muscle and joint pain. She had been diagnosed with fibromyalgia five years prior, and none of the ten different medications prescribed to her gave her any symptom relief. She had seen at least four different doctors and had undergone extensive blood work which was all "normal." Janice had lost all hope of improvement by the time I met her. "You are my last hope."

Janice appeared to be healthy, took no prescription medications, and had no known health problems. She had completed high school, married her high school sweetheart, and had three children who were now aged nine, twelve, and sixteen. Janice explained that she endured a relatively tough childhood and described herself as someone who "found it hard to be happy." She told me that she was constantly tired, depressed, and cold. She found it very challenging to be a stay at home mother... cooking, cleaning, and driving the kids from one activity to the next. She said that often after she would drop the children off at school, she would go back home and sleep for two or three more hours.

Janice explained that her muscle pain had started after the birth of her second child. Initially, her only other symptom was fatigue. Since that time, she had also developed irregular periods, insomnia, complete intolerance to stress, and depression. She was having difficulty losing her post-pregnancy weight, and her sugar cravings were at times unbearable. Over the course of the past ten years, she had been given prescription anti-depressants, sleeping pills, weight loss medications, and anti-inflammatory drugs. None of them helped and some caused side effects. At one point, her physician suggested she see a psychiatrist to which she responded, "I am not crazy, I am in pain."

Like many others who are not receiving relief from conventional medicine, Janice embarked on her own journey of self-diagnosis and self-healing. She spent thousands of dollars on self-help books, over-the-counter medications, herbal preparations and supplements from online companies. After conducting her own research, Janice was convinced that she suffered from adrenal fatigue because the description of her symptoms mirrored what she read in the book. Unfortunately, when she tried discussing this with other physicians, they would laugh or admonish her by saying, "there's no such thing as adrenal fatigue." Janice tried some supplements specifically designed to help and explained to me that some of them actually did make her feel somewhat better, though her symptoms were never completely resolved.

My take? Janice truly suffered from many of the expected symptoms of abnormally low daytime cortisol, including: chronic fatigue, fibromyalgia, stress sensitivity, and low-grade depression. In fact, her salivary cortisol pattern confirmed a flattened pattern of cortisol release during the daytime and a paradoxical rise in her late night cortisol reading.

Indeed she did have hypocortisolism, but an additional diagnostic work-up was critical to find out why these symptoms were occurring. After our initial meeting, a series of tests conducted, I found that Janice suffered from multiple vitamin deficiencies, particularly in vitamin C and the B vitamins, all of which are very important in the function of the adrenal glands. This was partially due to her unhealthy diet which was laden with sugar and caffeine, both of which strain the stress response system. In

LENA D. EDWARDS MD, FAARM

fact, when we looked at her saliva test results, her second collection (done around noon) showed a small rise in cortisol. Clearly, she did not have adrenal fatigue. If she did, her adrenal glands would have been incapable of making cortisol in response to the caffeine she drank all morning to stay awake.

Janice's fibromyalgia was coming from multiple sources. Her low cortisol was one, her nutritional deficiencies were another, and her insomnia was yet another. Because Janice's stress hormones were out of whack, none of her other hormones were working correctly either, her thyroid hormone being a primary example. She was like the many other people who are always told their thyroid lab test results are "in range," but they still exhibit numerous symptoms of low thyroid (functional hypothyroidism). Remember, if you have a fatigued stress response system (low HPA axis function), your body will shunt resources in the direction of survival.

At Janice's second visit, we outlined her initial treatment plan. I explained to her that her improvement would be gradual and that all aspects of her current lifestyle would need to be modified.

1.) She would need daily "down time" from her duties as a homemaker and mother. During this time, she could engage in activities she enjoyed.

2.) Janice was instructed to improve her diet and was given specifics on how to do so.

3.) She would keep a sleep journal. By scheduling specific sleep and wake times, avoiding naps, and utilizing such things as melatonin and magnesium at bedtime, Janice's "sleep hygiene" would improve.

4.) She began to do Pilates three days a week and would gradually increase the number of days she participated in the activity as her symptoms improved.

5.) Vitamin and mineral replacement were prescribed specific to her deficiencies and symptoms.

6.) Janice was prescribed a supplement containing plant adaptogens and a supplement containing grandulars. (see Chapter Nine)

I also explained to her that in addition to identifying and removing physical and psychological stressors, we would also need to continue to rule out any other underlying internal problems that could fuel her low cortisol state. Janice followed my advice, though it was difficult to schedule in a healthy lifestyle with three children in tow. Nonetheless, after six months, Janice reported feeling, "much happier, more confident, and physically and mentally refreshed."

CHRONIC PAIN SYNDROMES

Similar to the chronic pain syndrome of fibromyalgia, many other chronic pain conditions are resistant to currently available pain medications. This is problematic when you consider that one in ten adults suffer from chronic pain at some point in their lives. Chronic pain can blemish an otherwise happy existence by limiting a person's mobility, disrupting their relationships, and causing a loss of employment due to physical restrictions. This can lead to an increase in psychiatric illnesses, primarily depression. For our society, the economic burden inflicted by chronic pain syndromes is enormous, and current estimates suggest that, in terms of both lost productivity and treatment, the cost to U.S. society alone surpasses $100 billion annually.

It has been speculated that hypocortisolism is an important factor in mediating the effect of long term stress on chronic pain syndromes. Indeed, **studies have found patients with chronic low back pain, chronic pelvic pain, migraine and tension-type headache, and chronic facial pain to have co-existing hypocortisolism**. In several of these studies, patients with chronic pain syndromes have a higher incidence of physical and sexual abuse compared to the general population. And yet again, adrenal fatigue has not been found to be the cause. Rather, the brain's over-sensitivity to cortisol triggers an over-zealous "brake response" to cortisol production. Furthermore, when cortisol is away, inflammation comes out to play, and inflammation equals more pain.

MOOD DISORDERS

While some mood disorders, like Attention Deficit and Hyperactivity Disorder, bipolar disorder and some types of depression (as described in

Chapter Seven), are thought to be caused by high cortisol, other mood disorders can be brought on by low cortisol states.

- Atypical depression
- Seasonal depression
- Post traumatic stress disorder (PTSD)
- Fear of negative social evaluation ('rejection sensitivity')
- Cognitive vulnerability to depression
- Increase in somatoform disorders (symptoms without an identifiable cause)

Among these, the strongest correlation has been in the case of PTSD in which extreme stress induces a maladaptive stress response. Patients with PTSD typically experience high stress sensitivity, tension, increased excitability, and thought "intrusions." One 2004 study performed in Bosnian war refugees found that those with PTSD showed blunted morning cortisol responses compared to their non-PTSD counterparts. Several other studies of PTSD patients have also shown decreased cortisol levels to exist in Vietnam veterans, Holocaust survivors, and sexually abused women.

AUTOIMMUNE DISEASE

In the face of hypocortisolism, the "pro-inflammatory" side of your immune system is no longer under the suppressive influences of cortisol. Essentially, the parent is no longer around to guide the children. Unsupervised, these cells and chemical mediators cause destruction of your own tissues in the form of various autoimmune diseases. Some researchers actually believe that autoimmune diseases *may be caused by hypocortisolism.*

The following autoimmune diseases have been associated with low cortisol states:

- Rheumatoid arthritis
- Juvenile idiopathic (unknown cause) arthritis
- Dermatitis (skin inflammation)
- Type I diabetes
- Multiple sclerosis
- Autoimmune thyroid disease
- Allergic immune responses

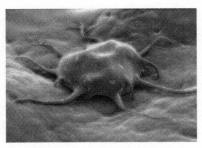

CANCER

With over a hundred different types of cancer in existence and 7.4 million deaths worldwide attributed to cancers, this disease affects almost everyone on the planet. And, while we certainly cannot fully "blame" low cortisol states on the onset of cancer (genetics, environmental toxins, and lifestyle play important roles), **hypocortisolism can be a factor in cancer development**, as you can see from the stats below.

- Hypocortisolism is altered in up to 30 percent of patients with **colorectal cancer** and if present, tolerance to chemotherapy and how well the treatment works may be adversely affected.
- **Breast cancer** patients with hypocortisolism may experience more severe disease, greater likelihood of their cancer spreading, and earlier death.
- **Ovarian cancer** patients with hypocortisolism experience more depression, poor physical sense of well-being, and more pronounced fatigue.
- Cancer patients with flattened cortisol patterns may not derive the full benefit from chemotherapy treatment. In fact, there is a large body of research on **cancer chrono-therapy**, the study of how circadian rhythm affects drug therapy and DNA repair in cancer cells and optimal timing of chemotherapy administration.

AND LAST BUT NOT LEAST...

As if what we have already discussed were not enough, our discussion would not be complete without adding a few more conditions which have been associated with hypocortisolism.

- Atherosclerosis (thickened artery walls)
- Functional bowel disease (Irritable bowel syndrome)
- Vital exhaustion (unusual fatigue)
- Asthma

　　　　　LENA D. EDWARDS MD, FAARM

- Allergies

IN A NUTSHELL:

This is a lot of information to digest. **Here are the important messages on hypocortisolism:**

1.) Hypocortisolism may be present in otherwise healthy individuals living under chronic stressful situations.

2.) Hypocortisolism is often seen in patients with stress-related bodily disorders such as CFS, FM, and PTSD, asthma, chronic pain syndromes, and autoimmune diseases.

3.) The ways in which low cortisol states arise are complex and multi-dimensional. Studies do not support the existence of adrenal fatigue. Rather, poor communication circuits between the brain and adrenal glands, tissue insensitivity, and/or hormone receptor malfunction are more often to blame.

4.) Genetic and developmental factors contribute to presence and extent of hypocortisolism. Due to the absence of cortisol's protective properties, low cortisol states make patients susceptible to the developing many stress-related bodily disorders and immune related diseases.

ARM YOURSELF WITH KNOWLEDGE

I want to urge you again, whether you're facing chronic pain, feeling the effects of depression or just plain worn-out from day-to-day life, **please work with your physician or healthcare provider to find out the "why" behind your symptoms**. Make it your goal to ensure that the proper tests are done and the results analysed in the correct way. Use your new found understanding of the issues to ask pointed questions. Arm yourself with additional knowledge.

And now that you are equipped with the knowledge of the problem, we are now finally ready to discuss the solutions. In the next chapter, we will expound upon the stress busting techniques you can use to "outsmart" your stress so that you can live a longer, more fulfilling and healthier life.

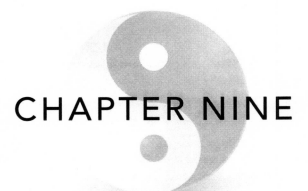

CHAPTER NINE

Taking Control: Outsmart Stress Before It Outsmarts You

"Every human being is the author of his own health or disease."

Buddha

Congratulations! You've reached the pinnacle of *Adrenalogic*. I've saved these "gems," the solutions, until the end because you now have a much better understanding of the stress response system and all of its wonderful complexities. In light of this, it's time to share the most beneficial evidence-based methods to outsmart stress and "live your best life," as Oprah Winfrey so often says.

Have you heard the expression, "nothing good comes easy?" If so, it serves as an intelligent reminder that good health takes effort. It must be attended to every day. With that said, I want to provide a quick primer (or reminder) on what <u>not</u> to do before we get into the essentials on supporting and encouraging optimal health.

LENA D. EDWARDS MD, FAARM

HABITS THAT STRESS YOUR STRESS RESPONSE SYSTEM

I'll be the first to admit that the relentless "get healthy" diatribes we're bombarded with can become annoying. Boat loads of statistics spew forth at us touting how the rates of depression and obesity continue their annual steep rate of incline.

So what? You may feel like it's someone else's problem and it doesn't apply to you. Well, it may not now, but it will. Your body is much more forgiving than any modern day machinery you choose to abuse, but at some unpredictable point, you will step into a disease land mine from which you will not be so easily rescued.

If you smoke, drink excessive amounts of alcohol, consume unhealthy food, and consider going back and forth to the refrigerator a valid exercise routine, then *stop*! No matter how many prescription medications and supplements you take to alleviate stress or mask symptoms, **nothing you do will ever make you feel better if you do not clean your proverbial internal house**.

I absolutely do not advocate for a "feast or famine" regime when it comes to healthy living; some of our "not so healthy" behaviors do serve other important purposes in our lives. As an example, good food and good wine are often very important social and bonding activities. In the United States, we eat when people are born, when people get married, for every major holiday, and when people die. So, it is irrational to say that you can never "cheat." Every once in a while is expected and acceptable as long as the majority of the time you honor your body with the gift of moderation.

SMOKING

For the 46.6 million American cigarette smokers reading this, you already know that the "cancer sticks" you find difficult to give up put a very large bulls-eye on your back. And no, it is not just the nicotine. As per information from the Center for Disease Control and Prevention: direct and second-hand smoke also results in the ingestion of nearly 4,000 chemicals.

As we have already discussed, smoking cigarettes raises cortisol – one of the very outcomes we're trying to avoid. Quitting any habit, especially smoking, can be difficult. But any behavior that is learned can be unlearned given the right attitude and environment. The Center for Disease Control offers some very helpful tips on how to quit smoking which include identifying why you smoke and why you want to quit, not setting unrealistic expectations for yourself, and getting help if you need it.

SLEEP

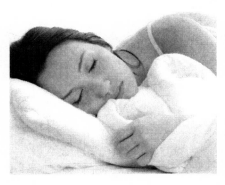

Do you work third shift or stay up late each night surfing the web or watching TV? While being a "night owl" may seem harmless enough, proper sleep hygiene is one key to good health and diminished stress levels. Recall our discussions earlier about the effects of shift work and sleep deprivation? The International Agency for Research on Cancer (IARC) has concluded that "shift work that involves circadian disruption" is considered a Group 2A carcinogen and "probably carcinogenic to humans." That's major news. In simple terms it means that continuous work involving shifts which disrupt normal sleep patterns can contribute to cancer development.

And what of the term good "sleep hygiene" to which I've referenced throughout the book? It's a fancy term which is meant to simply convey a well-ordered, healthy sleep routine. If you have trouble sleeping or feel like your sleep routine could use an overhaul, keep these points in mind:

- **Identify secondary causes** (drugs, foods, sleep apnea, pets, etc.)
- **Behavioral modification is essential** (no watching television, exercising, working on your computer, or cleaning your house before bedtime)
- **Adopt a regular and consistent sleep wake cycle** (remember your hormones are released in direct relation to your sleep/wake cycle)

LENA D. EDWARDS MD, FAARM

- **Employ stress reduction techniques** (meditation, guided imagery, quite reading, deep breathing)
- **Avoid prescription sleep aides and alcohol** (they are Band-Aid solutions that can ultimately cause side effects including addiction)
- **Use your bedroom for sleep and intimacy only**
- **Avoid third shift work if at all possible.** If this is not an option, consider adding melatonin and do your best to maintain a regular sleep/wake cycle even on the days you do not work.

WEIGHT

Are you in the group of people who is always on a diet but never losing weight? Well, your body fat percentage is directly tied to how you feel, what diseases you may develop, and how early in life you may die.

For those of you who are misinformed about weight and its effects, it is not just what one puts in their mouth that determines their body weight. Hormones, intestinal health, sleep patterns, genetics, exercise patterns, and food allergies are only some of the things that contribute. The dieting industry is a billion dollar industry for two main reasons:

1.) People want a quick fix

2.) Behaviors are hard to change

I'm not talking down to you here, I can tell you from experience that those radical diets never work! In fact, I too have struggled with obesity and found that maintaining a healthy weight involved making gradual changes, setting realistic expectations, keeping a positive mental attitude, and keeping an "overweight" picture of myself on my refrigerator to prevent me from finding solace in food when faced with another emotional crisis.

If you currently indulge in a health-threatening habits, I encourage you to educate yourself, conduct research, talk to your healthcare professional, and take the steps necessary to overcome these bad habits now before they overcome you.

HEALTHY HABITS THAT "OUTSMART" STRESS

Before you begin your journey towards self-awareness, health and well-being, you must first consider two important things:

1.) **Your life is a marathon, not a race.** You did not arrive at your current location overnight. Therefore give yourself time to implement new habits and actions.

2.) **Identify the reason(s) why you are in your current place in life.**

A key point: Discuss any concerns with your doctor and, armed with the information you've gained here, take a stand. Don't become one of the 50 percent of Americans who accepts a prescription drug to suppress or disguise your symptoms. Early identification can only happen by understanding that a statistical "norm" is not the same as optimal health. This will allow for early treatment and resolution of your symptoms so you can get back to living your life.

GET PREPARED

You will do yourself (and your healthcare provider) a great service if you prepare for your first visit:

1.) **Identify and eliminate stressors** over which you have control. This can range from very easy (i.e. tidying your room every day and avoiding fast food) to rather difficult (i.e. leaving a troubled relationship or getting sober).

There is always help available whether through friends, family, a crisis line, a non-profit group, a church, or an online support group.

2.) **Consider adjusting your attitude** to personal stressors. Whether alone or through "talk therapy," a better understanding of why you feel the way you do allows you to begin to understand patterns and modify behavior. It can also mean that you learn to become more self-confident in your decisions and opinions.

3.) **Embrace exercise.** I suggest to you that if you have enough time to sit in rush hour traffic or watch television, you can spare at least thirty minutes a day to exercise. Our bodies were not designed to be sedentary, and the health benefits of exercise have been shown time and time again. If you have been on the couch for a while, start with low impact exercises, yoga or Pilates. These types of exercise have been shown to help people in all walks of life to de-stress, lose weight, maintain happiness, and prevent disease. We'll address the benefits of yoga later in this chapter.

4.) **Maintain a healthy body weight.** Excess body fat causes every disease in the book. More body fat means more inflammation which means more stress on your HPA axis.

5.) **Examine your spirituality/religiosity.** This means different things to different people and depends upon your upbringing, personal views, and degree of self-enlightenment. Suffice to say: research has shown that people who identify with a higher being or have a religious affiliation enjoy less stress, better health, and longer life spans.

6.) **Modify your diet.** The saying "you are what you eat" was coined for good reason. Your stress (and sex) hormones are profoundly influenced by what, how, and when you eat. I often tell my patients, "If nature didn't make it, then don't eat it." The more processed, fried, colored, and "chemicalized" the food you consume, the more stress it puts on your system. Eat good quality protein and complex carbohydrates in moderation and frequently throughout the day. For those of you on one of the many popular diets that severely restrict calories, give it up. Not only will your hormones hate you for it, you will gain back your weight (plus some) once you quit said diet. Over 70 percent of your body is water, so drink up. And finally, instead of super sizing your meal, supersize your energy by choosing not to pollute your body with junk food.

Let's take a look at what happens if you eat a diet high on the glycemic index (foods that disproportionately raise blood sugar):

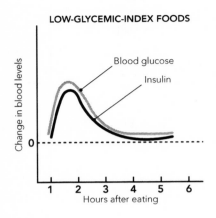

LOW-GLYCEMIC-INDEX FOODS

Change in blood levels

Blood glucose
Insulin

0

1 2 3 4 5 6
Hours after eating

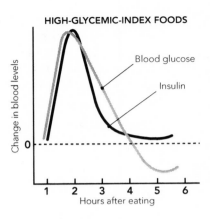

HIGH-GLYCEMIC-INDEX FOODS

Change in blood levels

Blood glucose
Insulin

0

1 2 3 4 5 6
Hours after eating

You will see how eating foods that significantly raise your blood sugar like candy, potatoes, pasta, and white bread, can cause a spike in your insulin (and in your cortisol) at first. After several hours, your blood sugar will come crashing down to which your body responds by saying, "I need carbs and I need them now!" Eating healthy foods will stop this rollercoaster ride by keeping your glucose, insulin, and cortisol at even levels. You can also help to reduce the "glycemic load" of foods by eating them in combination with low glycemic index foods such as nuts, apples, berries, and legumes.

7.) **Meditate.** If you are a Type A personality like me, you may find sitting quietly, breathing deeply, and clearing your head of all thoughts almost impossible. However, if you read the medical literature on the health benefits of meditating, you may reconsider. We will discuss this further.

8.) **Get enough ZZZs.** Unless you want to feel like you once did when you were the parent of a newborn *forever* and shave about ten years off your life, you have to sleep. The recommended number of hours varies, since we typically require less sleep as we age. **A good rule of thumb is to shoot for around seven hours of uninterrupted sleep every night**. Identify and eliminate anything causing a disruption to your sleep. If your spouse snores,

LENA D. EDWARDS MD, FAARM

buy ear plugs or sleep in another room. Better yet, suggest they see their doctor for help. If your pets wake you or fuels your pet allergies, you may need to find another place for them to sleep. And, consider not eating foods heavily laden with sugar or drinking caffeine before bedtime. I once had a patient who complained of insomnia for over one year. Unfortunately, she neglected to tell me that she drank a caffeinated beverage every night as she read in bed. If simple lifestyle changes do not work, talk to your healthcare provider about non-prescription sleep aides such as melatonin, 5-HTP, phosphatidylserine, or inositol. Several of these are outlined in more detail below.

9.) **Learn to Relax.** In our "go, go, go" society, some people view relaxation as a sign of laziness or boredom. Well, your stress response system views it as highly therapeutic. Our bodies and brains need to decompress in order to work at optimal levels.

To supplement these basic points, let's take a closer look at some of the ways in which you can 'outsmart' your stress through exercise and nutritional supplementation.

YOGA AND MEDITATION MAKE YOUR HPA AXIS HAPPY

We have already discussed how stress and chronic HPA axis abnormalities can cause aging. But for many, *quality* is more valuable than *quantity*. The mind has profound power over our quality of life. Another one of those clichés that rings true: "mind over matter." Chronic stress, over-stimulation, inflated expectations, and mental anguish strain our brains, drain our energy, and reduce our capacity to enjoy our lives. Mind-body practices such as yoga, meditation, and imagery promote a sense of peace and serenity which allows one to be fully present, happy, and healthy.

You may already know that in many countries such as India, yoga and meditation are practiced daily – sometimes multiple times per day. Meditation allows the body to fully engage and relax, centering us and often bringing peace and insight – an opportunity not available to us when we're racing around from sun-up to sundown. Research on meditation has been done since the early 1960's, but the study of yoga and breathing practices has come about much more recently.

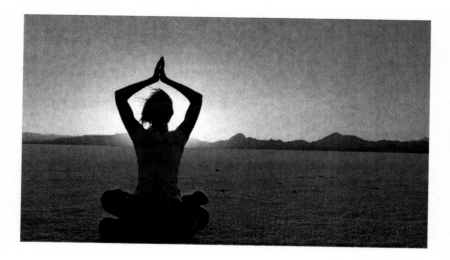

Yoga is a 5000 year-old philosophy whose basic premise is that there is a relationship between the mind and the breath that allows one to affect their mind and consciousness by manipulating the way they breathe. The practice of deep breathing is believed to eliminate toxic substances, to clear "negative air," to increase oxygen levels, and to improve "positive energy," all of which strengthen the mind and the body.

The philosophy of these practices considers **the biggest stress to come from distress of one's mind as it oscillates between things it wants and things it doesn't.** This is what happens when we dwell on past mistakes or worry about something that hasn't even happened yet. If you saw the movie *Kung Fu Panda*, you remember the wise turtle Ooguay telling the panda, "Yesterday is history, tomorrow is a mystery, but today is a gift. That is why it is called the 'present'."

But exactly how do mindful practices bring about less stress and improved health? The medical literature suggests it is from the positive influences on the HPA axis. Research has shown yoga and meditation can:

LENA D. EDWARDS MD, FAARM

- Reduce stress induced cortisol secretion
- Reduce inflammation
- Improve cortisol release patterns
- Improve HPA axis regulation
- Improve the quality of life and stress tolerance in breast and prostate cancer survivors by improving cortisol release patterns and reducing inflammation
- Reduce the risk of heart disease in postmenopausal women
- Positively impact patients with inflammatory bowel disease
- Improve mood and anxiety better than a similar walking exercise

EMBRACE ADAPTOGENS

What exactly is an *adaptogen* and how can it help you? As it name probably implies, an adaptogen is **a compound that increases one's ability to adapt to and avoid damage (stress, trauma, fatigue, etc.) from environmental stressors.** The numerous health benefits of adaptogens have been realized in Ayurvedic (traditional Indian) and Chinese medicine for thousands of years, but scientific research on these plant derived substances only began in the 1940's.

Plant adaptogens essentially induce a state of 'beneficial stress' in an attempt to teach your stress response to behave itself; this is similar to what moderate exercise does. If you have an over-stimulated HPA axis, adaptogens help to tone that down. If your HPA axis is in the gutter, adaptogens help to lift it up. Their ultimate effect is *maintenance of homeostasis* (establishing balance). Adaptogens have also been shown to have favorable effect on your immune systems which you now know is profoundly tied to your stress response system.

The following is a partial listing of some of the plant adaptogens that have been identified and/or studied in relation to healing and maintaining a healthy HPA axis:

- Ashwaganda *(Withania somnifera)*
- Rhodiola (*Rhodiola rosea*, also known as Artic Root or Golden Root)
- Panax Ginseng
- Korean ginseng

- Licorice *(Glycyrrhiza glabra)*
- Cordyceps *(Cordyceps sinensis)*
- Noni *(Morinda citrifolia)*
- Maca *(Lepidium perumianum)*
- Holy Basil *(Ocimum Sanctum)*
- Bacopa (also known as water hyssop)
- Schisandra *(Schisandra chinensis)*
- Astragalus (also known as locoweed)
- Siberian Ginseng *(Eleutherococcus sneticosus)*

Each one of these plant adaptogens has hundreds or even thousands of subspecies, so you can see how complicated it can be. Suffice to say that each group has been shown to have specific properties and potential health benefits. We will focus on some of the beneficial effects of those more heavily researched.

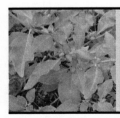

ASHWAGANDA
- Stimulates thyroid function
- Protects the brain and heart
- Completely safe, no side effects
- Neutralizes free radicals
- Favorable effects on immune system

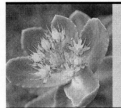

RHODIOLA
- Improves mental performance and brain function
- Improves stress induced mental and physical fatigue
- Improves physical endurance
- Anti-oxidant and anti-cancer and anti-inflammatory

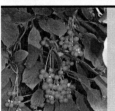

SCHISANDRA
- Increases physical work capacity and endurance
- Improves mental function, mental capacity, and mental accuracy
- Reduces fatigue, muscle pain, shortness of breath after extreme physical activity
- Beneficial in mood disorders and many gastrointestinal diseases

LENA D. EDWARDS MD, FAARM

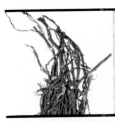

LICORICE
- Increases cortisol levels
- Improves mood and memory
- Indirect improvement in immune system function
- Anti-fungal, anti-viral, anti-ulcer

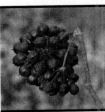

SIBERIAN GINSENG
- Prevent/treat herpes simplex II infections
- Improve memory
- Improve physical endurance and body strength
- Lowers cholesterol, improves anxiety
- Improves visual perception

Many companies now manufacture supplements containing varied combinations of two or more adaptogens plus or minus a few other ingredients. I strongly **encourage you to work with your healthcare provider before consuming any adaptogenic product** to ensure it is the correct one for you. You should also purchase only high quality, **pharmaceutical grade products**. Since the FDA does not regulate the supplement industry in the U.S, it is very easy to get a supplement that is contaminated, unreliable, or even dangerous. A knowledgeable integrative healthcare provider can also guide you since their broad knowledge base of all plant adaptogens will allow them to educate you about potential side effects and possible drug/herb interactions.

REMEMBER YOUR A-B-Cs

My patients often ask me why it is necessary for them to take vitamins and minerals. Their question is always, "Shouldn't the food I eat give me everything I need?" That is a legitimate question, and my answer to them is: "Ideally, yes." I then throw a simple trivia question their way: What do chronic stress, unhealthy diets filled with processed foods, undiagnosed food allergies, alcohol, prescription drugs, and unhealthy bowels all have in common? Answer: They all cause nutrient malabsorption. On the flip side, I have other patients who believe their over the-counter multiple vitamin pill covers all the bases. Wrong again.

The next time you are buying a bottle of vitamins, look at the label. It looks great, right? 100 percent of the recommended daily intake (RDI) for one vitamin and 200 percent of the RDI of another. How can you possibly go wrong? Remember our discussion of the terms "sufficient" and "optimal" from Chapter Five when we were discussing lab testing? Well, we can essentially have the same conversation when it comes to vitamin supplementation. You, your lifestyle and health habits, and your stress levels are individually unique to you. How can one generic multi-vitamin be appropriate for you, your forty-five-year-old husband, and your eighteen-year-old daughter?

There are a number of excellent books on vitamins and nutrients, so I am not going to delve into the subject here. What I am going to do is to discuss with you some of the vitamins and minerals that are especially important in maintaining a healthy HPA axis. Keep in mind that doses have not been provided because they will vary based upon a number of individual factors. This is where your doctor can step in and help out.

VITAMIN C
Your adrenal glands contain the highest concentration of Vitamin C in your body. Vitamin C is absolutely essential in maintaining not only optimal cortisol levels but catecholamine levels as well. During periods of stress, your adrenal glands release their Vitamin C stores. Why?

During periods of stress when ACTH causes a rise in cortisol, the adrenal glands release their stores of Vitamin C. The Vitamin C released locally within the adrenal glands causes the blood vessels to dilate thereby allowing for more cortisol production and release to meet the increased demand. Chronic stress can lead to depletion of adrenal Vitamin C stores.

Excellent food sources of Vitamin C are most fruits and vegetables.

MAGNESIUM
Magnesium is perhaps one of the most vital minerals in that it is involved in over three hundred enzyme pathways in your body. Its primary function is in cell function and energy transfer. Other important functions of magnesium are:

- Improves insulin sensitivity and blood sugar control
- Improves levels of growth hormone and melatonin during sleep
- Improves pain control
- Maintains muscle and nerve function
- Maintains a healthy immune system

Magnesium deficiency results in a stress effect and increased susceptibility to internal damage produced by stress. Stress induced magnesium supplementation has been shown to prevent a rise in ACTH (hence cortisol) during sleep, which is why it is recommended by many integrative medical practitioners as a sleep aide. Supplementation also prevents an excessive rise in cortisol after exercise. Magnesium can also be calming and help to correct aggression and anxiety. Foods rich in magnesium are almonds, spinach, soybeans, cashews, and halibut. Your doctor can guide you on the appropriate type and dose of magnesium should supplementation be necessary.

B VITAMINS

Vitamin B1, otherwise known as thiamine, is important in maintaining proper nerve and heart function as well as helping your body to metabolize sugars in your diet. Thiamine is found in a wide variety of food sources such as pork, oatmeal, sunflower seeds, and unprocessed whole grains. As such, it is unusual to be deficient in this vitamin unless you have a very restricted diet, have an eating disorder, or are an alcoholic.

Thiamine has been found to possess another outstanding quality: it may help prevent hypercortisolism. In fact, a Russian study found that surgical patients treated with thiamine experienced a less pronounced stress-induced rise in cortisol both during and after surgery Through the positive results of this and other clinical studies, the authors recommended that thiamine could be an effective remedy for "adrenal gland protection" from the profound stress induced by surgery.

Vitamin B6, or pyridoxal, is even more amazing when it comes to protecting your stress response system. Normally it is used by your body in the production of various neurotransmitters and histamine as well as serving as an important cofactor in numerous other processes. But, research has shown pyridoxal to do some interesting things when it comes to maintaining normal HPA axis function including aiding pregnancy-induced hypercortisolism and improving rhythmic control of the HPA axis.

Finally, **Vitamin B5**, or pantothene, supplementation has been shown to improve cortisol balance in a variety of human conditions. Although nearly every food has some amount of Vitamin B5, higher levels are found in whole grains, legumes, avocados, and yogurt.

HERBS, AMINO ACIDS, AND OTHERS
If your conventional medicine doctor rolls his eyes when you mention the word "herb," you can open *Adrenalogic* to this page and enlighten him. A global company far better than any pharmaceutical company has already created solutions to nearly all human ailments. The company name? Mother Nature. Although there are numerous beneficial substances out there, we are now going to focus on some of the more well studied herbs and amino acids an unhappy stress response system longs for.

THEANINE
Theanine is an amino acid derived from the leaves of green tea. It works within the body to increase alpha brain wave activity, the calming waves your brain emits when you are in a relaxed state of alertness as when meditating. Theanine has also been shown to: counteract the stimulating effects of caffeine, lower LDL (bad) cholesterol, and prevent cortisol levels from getting too high when you are in high stress situations. Even more amazing, Theanine has been shown to protect the brain from stroke induced brain damage.

Theanine is essentially nature's form of the drug Xanax, working quickly without the high or the side effects. I actually have several patients who frequent my office around holiday season to buy bottles of Theanine as stocking stuffers. You will be happy to know that Theanine is essentially free of side effects and does not interact with any supplement or medication. Judy, our college student from Chapter One, experienced excellent results using Theanine. It helped her stay calm but not groggy during her stressful day, protected her stress response system from all the caffeine she was drinking to stay awake, and helped shut her mind off at bedtime.

PHOSPHATIDYLSERINE (PS)

This is one of those lengthy scientific terms that may make you turn the page so we call it "PS" instead. Phosphatidylserine is an amino acid important in the communication and activity of our brain cells. Research has shown that when PS is given as a supplement, it may have several beneficial effects:

- It can protect overstimulation of the HPA axis thereby preventing surges in cortisol
- It results in a decrease in post-exercise cortisol levels and improves mood and muscle soreness that sometimes occur after overtraining
- It raises the levels of calming neurotransmitters, such as dopamine, thereby improving mood
- It may prevent chronic stress induced memory loss

Recall our business executive from Chapter Seven, Jason, a poster child for hypercortisolism? I prescribed low dose PS in the morning to prevent him from self-combusting, and higher doses at night to help him sleep. Worked like a charm!

5-HYDROXYTRYTOPHAN (5-HTP)

5-HTP is a derivative of the amino acid tryptophan... you know, the hormone in potatoes and turkey that make you calm and tired (probably the reason these foods are a mainstay at Thanksgiving)? This is one of the supplements I also prescribed for Jason to help his mood and sleep. 5-HTP is a middle step between tryptophan and two very important hormones, serotonin and melatonin. So, if you are low on 5-HTP, you are moody but never "in the mood," sleepy because you can't sleep, and hungry because you can't get full.

TRYPTOPHAN → 5-HTP → SEROTONIN → MELATONIN

Since 5-HTP helps sleep and mood, it is easy to see how it can be helpful in treating several aspects of abnormal HPA axis function. Here are a few tidbits you may find quite interesting: **90 - 95 percent of your serotonin is made in your intestines not your brain**, and **vitamins B3 and B6 are**

very important cofactors in serotonin production. Keep this in mind because your doctor should also be evaluating your intestinal health and supplementing B-vitamins if you complain of symptoms of HPA axis dysfunction.

DHEA

We have already discussed DHEA and its potential role in treating such conditions as osteoporosis, rheumatoid arthritis, and insulin resistance. But also remember that DHEA is cortisol's nemesis. In hypercortisol patients who are stressed and wired, taking a DHEA supplement can help to bring cortisol levels down and protect your brain and other tissues from its damaging effects.

Even though DHEA is a hormone, it is available over the counter without a prescription. This is concerning, in part, because of DHEA's ability to transform into other hormones, mainly testosterone and estrogen. Also, because it is touted to promote energy levels, people with low cortisol may take it thinking they have found their cure... Bad idea! If your already low cortisol is put in the ring with the DHEA heavyweight, your cortisol is going down!

I would strongly advise you to use DHEA, and Pregnenolone, another adrenal gland hormone available over the counter, only under the supervision of a knowledgeable healthcare provider. I have seen far too many patients do more harm than good after taking these supplements, especially in the wrong doses.

OTHER TOOLS IN THE STRESS RELIEF TOOL BOX

- **Tyrosine**
  - Precursor to catecholamines
  - Improve mood and memory
  - Reduce effects of stress on performance
- **Plant sterols**
  - Increases DHEA
  - Maintains normal cortisol levels and HPA axis balance during exercise

- **GABA**
  - Anti-anxiety
  - Promotes relaxation and sleep
  - Reduces markers of stress
- **Melatonin**
  - Maintains normal circadian sleep/wake cycle
  - Prevents HPA axis overactivation
  - Potent anti-oxidant

GLANDULARS

Glandulars are preparations containing various combinations of adrenal, hypothalamus, pituitary, and/or thyroid gland elements, usually from bovine (cow) or porcine (pig) sources. They were invented and made commercially available in the early 1930's and heavily researched in the 1940's in the treatment of tuberculosis, diabetes, psoriasis, and other inflammatory conditions. Once steroid drugs like cortisone became available, enthusiasm over glandulars fizzled out.

The basic idea behind using glandulars is that by giving an extract of an organ similar to the one that is functioning at a sub-par level, the function of the "lazy" or "exhausted" gland will improve. Glandulars are sort of like your personal trainer cheering you on as you cry in pain. Unless a person has an allergy to beef or pork, these supplements are relatively safe and do not shut down the body's own hormone when used appropriately in low doses. They are not recommended as the sole treatment for HPA axis dysfunction or as alternatives to standard medical treatment. Again, even though they are available over the counter, buyer beware.

PHARMACOLOGIC AGENTS

While I no longer immediately reach for my prescription pad for every patient ailment, there is a place for prescription drug therapy in the treatment of some stress related diseases. We will discuss two examples below.

HYDROCORTISONE

Hydrocortisone (HC) is a steroid with low potency with actions similar to those of our bodies' own cortisol. Although typically believed to only benefit patients with complete cortisol deficiency (Addison's Disease), patients with very flat cortisol release patterns, such as those with chronic fatigue syndrome, fibromyalgia, and those who are critically ill may benefit from the addition of low dose hydrocortisone to their treatment regimens.

My patients often become quite concerned when I prescribe low dose HC, and I have to spend extra time explaining how it is different from some of the more potent steroids like Prednisone. I always forewarn them of the drug insert they will receive which may horrify them as they read the list of side effects of other steroids, namely bone loss, immune system suppression, adrenal gland suppression, and weight gain. Low dose HC used short term does not typically cause these side effects. In fact, some studies have shown that low dose HC may actually help improve immune system function. Consider it the same as a business hiring part-time help during the Christmas season so the full-time employees don't quit from overwork and exhaustion.

If you are suffering from CFS or FM or any condition in which you are experiencing profound fatigue in the face of very low daytime cortisol levels, discuss adding low dose HC with your doctor to complement the other treatment modalities you are prescribed.

FLUDROCORTISONE
Remember our brief discussion of the adrenal gland hormone aldosterone? Well, fludrocortisone (FC) mimics the action of aldosterone in the body - namely fluid and sodium retention and balancing potassium. Because of its actions, side effects of FC can include high blood pressure, fluid retention, headaches, and low potassium.

If you have ever suffered through the agony of orthostatic hypotension (dizziness and fluctuating blood pressure and pulse), your doctor may have prescribed this medication. In this condition, your blood pressure and pulse are not properly regulated, and you may feel heart palpitations, dizziness, or actually pass out. This condition may actually be quite common in patients with low cortisol states as we discussed earlier. Most often, FC is used only temporarily as other causes of the problem are identified and treated.

An entire book could be written on the contents in this chapter alone. However, these are the highlights which offer the best tools to keep your HPA axis balanced and healthy. I urge you to utilize these tools to regain your health and vitality. Find a healthcare provider who has been properly trained to thoroughly understand stress, HPA axis dysfunction, and the treatment options thereof. Be an active participant in this process, ask questions, and offer suggestions. Remember the doctor is your team-mate, not your parent. Share this information with friends, family members, coworkers, and others so that they too can benefit and take steps to improve their health.

1. List the top ten most stressful aspects of your life. Are there potential solutions or alternatives?

_____

_____

_____

_____

_____

_____

_____

_____

_____

_____

2. What are five or more realistic stress busting options that you can incorporate into your daily, weekly, or monthly routine?

_____

_____

_____

_____

_____

_____

_____

_____

3. List five or more positive influences or aspects of your life that you can turn to or focus on when you are stressed out?

_____

_____

_____

_____

_____

_____

_____

_____

LENA D. EDWARDS MD, FAARM

4. Make a list of 25 things you are grateful for.

_____

_____

_____

_____

_____

_____

_____

_____

_____

_____

_____

_____

_____

_____

_____

_____

_____

_____

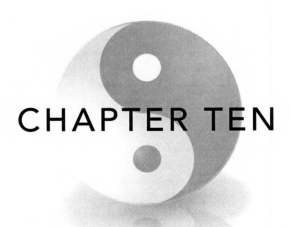

CHAPTER TEN

Words Of Wisdom - From Someone Who's Been There

"I've learned from experience that the greater part of our happiness or misery depends on our dispositions and not on our circumstances."

Martha Washington

By now, you may be experiencing a wave of different emotions: amazement, confusion, enlightenment, and perhaps even vindication. I can tell you the universal emotion expressed by my patients is hope – perhaps the most profoundly positive emotion one can feel.

While Western medicine has allowed us amazing advances in both diagnosis and treatment of disease, there is a "grey zone" that prevails: a gaping chasm in which prescription drugs may not be the answer. It is partially for this reason that people spend billions of dollars annually on nutritional supplements and self-help books to treat their own medical conditions, conditions that modern medicine may overlook. However, it appears the engine of "conventional medicine" may be losing steam at

LENA D. EDWARDS MD, FAARM

the hands of the millions of patients like you who feel bad and want to regain their health in a more proactive fashion.

To give you a better understanding of how I arrived at my current stance on treatment, I would like to share with you how some of my own experiences changed my life. Change can be very scary and often unwelcome but is inevitable. When I was in medical training, the most exciting me thing for me was the Eureka! moment when I saved a patient's life or diagnosed and treated someone who had a medical condition no one else could previously diagnose. Sure, tests and prescription medications were tools in my tool box, but the more important tools were *time and communication*. Unfortunately, as time went by and I entered private practice, the "art" of medicine was seemingly transformed into the business of medicine. I gradually felt that my roles as healer, scholar, and educator were being overtaken by my new roles as an administrator, accountant, and insurance agent. As the sole owner of my practice, I became too busy and financially strapped to engage in the practicing medicine the way I once had. It took dedication and perseverance to re-evaluate my priorities and restructure my life and my medical practice so as to regain the balance essential to my being a passionate healer and educator: the *time to communicate* with my patients. "Your patients will give you the diagnosis if you simply listen to them," one of my wise medical school instructors told me.

The light-switch clicked on when I aligned my two types of medical training. You see, my training in internal medicine taught me the *how* and the *what*, but my training in integrative and functional medicine taught me the *why*. The same medical picture now had more definition and depth because the angle of my lens had changed. Instead of trying to madly rush through an office visit, I now take the time to communicate with my patients. Instead of pulling out my prescription pad for ailments which often did not require drug treatment, I pull out the names of fitness clubs, meditation centers, counselors, health food stores, and nutritionists. At every patient's first visit, I outline my role as their health "co-director" and help them to understand that although I am there to medically guide them, they are responsible for making the healthy life choices essential for regaining their health and outsmarting their stress. My patients often ask me why I decided to, "quit practicing traditional internal medicine," and my response to them is, "Actually, I finally feel like I am practicing true internal medicine."

You may have read *Adrenalogic* appreciating the data but wondering, "How can this woman possibly understand what it is like for me? Sure, being a doctor is tough, but how does she know what it is like to be unemployed, uninsured, or in an unhealthy relationship?" Now, although this book is not an autobiography, I can assure you that indirectly it is. I could've written a book about anything, but I chose to write my first book on something very personal to me: *stress*. In fact, I rank my life experience right up there with my medical training as the most influential factors in defining the type of doctor and person I have become. Helping people understand stress, how it can either help them or slowly kill them, and how they can outsmart and overcome it has become my passion… My divine calling, if you will. Believe me, I know because I almost allowed my stress to outsmart me too.

As a Type A personality, I often find myself wearing many, many "hats." As such, in addition to my "doctor hat," I wear hats corresponding to my roles as mother, business owner, employer, employee, author, speaker, teacher, significant other, daughter, and sister. I'm not saying this so you can reach for your miniature violin and play a little rendition of "my heart bleeds for you." Rather, what I hope you to take away from this brief glimpse into my life is that *I understand*. I have personally and professionally "been there and done that" with just about everything you can think of. As such, I feel amply qualified to expertly guide you through these many pages.

I have had several unsettling life experiences just like everyone else, but there is one particularly memorable event that I would like to share with you. In 2003, I had a thriving practice with over two thousand patients. My hectic work schedule kept me distracted enough not to notice that my hair was falling out and my muscles were deteriorating. My diet consisted of crackers and soda from which my intestinal tract constantly begged for mercy. Because I clearly wasn't busy enough, I decided to add more to my plate by getting trained in other areas of medicine: Botox, mesotherapy, laser therapy, anti-aging, bio-identical hormone replacement, integrative medicine… it was never-ending. With all these additional services came hundreds more patients which my office couldn't contain. I decided to search for a new space and was approached by a seemingly charming real estate agent who suggested we purchase the building together – this move marked the beginning of the end for me.

It was in 2004 that I received the dreaded "wake-up "call which caused me to crash into the proverbial wall. Some may ignore these calls, and I tried to do the same. I received no hint of what was coming; if I had I might have been better prepared. This literal wake-up call notified me that my real estate partner had absconded with all of the mortgage payments and I was forced to file bankruptcy. I lost everything, including my medical practice, in the process. It was a devastating blow, but it didn't kill me. In fact, quite the opposite: for I can now appreciate the fact that losing my business probably saved my life instead. "How?," you may ask.

As you have probably gathered by now, you have a great deal of control over how a stressor affects you. And your perception becomes your reality which then fuels your reaction. Our *perceptions* to things can be as unique to us as our fingerprints and are also partially programmed into our DNA. Your surroundings and circumstances also play a significant role in how you react. For instance, before losing my business, I was a complete control freak. Everything had to be perfect, everything needed to be done yesterday, and there could never be room for error. My perception of life was that "average was the enemy of good." Well, pardon the cliché, but this life lesson gave me a new perspective: my perceptions and reactions to stressful situations were slowly killing me. And even though I believed I was in complete control over my life, it only took one event to completely change it! I was able to adapt to this devastating blow. Have you adapted from yours?

So for all the rest of you who have hit rock bottom at some point in your life and can empathize with my situation, I pose to you this question: how did you handle it? Did you "outsmart" it or did it outsmart you? Believe me, I went through the typical stages of grief and loss, but I always tried to remember that amplifying stress with more stress would never get me out of my emotional black hole. I'm human too, and I would be lying if

I said I did not falter along the way, but I've never lost sight of the ultimate goal... *Self-preservation*. Absolutely I considered leaving the practice of medicine to move to Hawaii and become a beach bum. Alcohol and other "emotional tranquilizers" were always an option over exercise and meditation, but I chose the healthier options. Negative thoughts like, "What have you done?!" echoed through my head every day, but I chose to ignore them. Instead of succumbing to short term Band-Aid solutions, I chose healthier long-term solutions by maintaining my body, sanity, and well-being through making positive choices.

I see thousands of patients a year, men and women of different ages, backgrounds, and professions. I listen very carefully to the details of their lives and always ask them about what "stresses them out." The patient's stressors and their reactions to them are often the very reason why they feel "bad" and come to see me. Because of my life experiences, my many hats now give me clarity to meet the *person* in front of me, not the patient. In fact, I may occasionally share bits of my personal experiences with them so they realize I know how it feels to be down, overweight, unemployed, uninsured, or whatever the life hit may be. **Here are some of Dr. Lena Edwards' words of wisdom for outsmarting stress:**

- Perfect the tone and proper application of the word, "**No**." Even though the word is small in size, it can be enormous in meaning. Use it as the moat around your castle. Feel empowered to say "no" whenever you feel it's reasonable to do so.
- A perfectly reasonable explanation to a question can be **"Because"**... You are unique in your thoughts, emotions, and perceptions. Sometimes an explanation is not always necessary.
- On some days, my motto is: **Be glad I showed up!** You can never be everything to everyone all the time. People in your life may occasionally forget this and will benefit from your gentle reminders.
- **The "higher power" may not always be available, so sometimes people will just have to deal with you.** Don't expect perfection, expect humanity. Sarcasm can occasionally be medicinal.
- **Put your heart on a diet.** Love in a manner that fosters growth and independence not control, worry, and fear. And love yourself

LENA D. EDWARDS MD, FAARM

first. If you've flown on a plane, you'll be familiar with the phrase, "adjust your oxygen mask first before assisting others." Use this as a metaphor when living your own life.

- Unlike your home and your car, **your body is irreplaceable**, so treat it well. Once health is lost, it is difficult to regain. How would you treat the body of your child?
- **Life happens, so let it.** You are profoundly important as a unique individual, but you too shall pass.
- **Be happy you woke up today.** Enough said.

I trust that my truthfulness has inspired you – or at least made you think. And, now that we've reached the book's conclusion, I truly hope that the information you have learned will have a positive and influential impact on your life. I feel that I have been offered a second chance to live life healthier and happier, and in gratitude, I wrote *Adrenalogic*. I wish you all the best in your journey towards a balanced life.

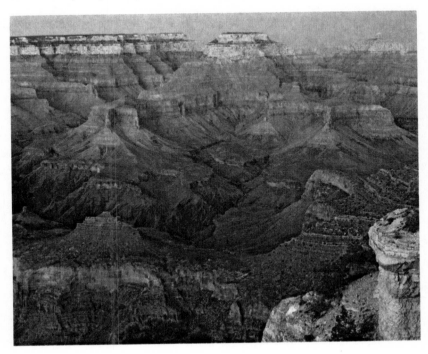

REFERENCES

CHAPTER ONE

Cannon WB. Bodily changes in pain, hunger, fear, and rage. New York: Appleton-Century-Crofts. 1929.

Goldstein DS, Kopin IJ. Evolution of concepts of stress. Stress. 2007 Jun; 10 (2) :109-20.

McEwen B. Protective and Damaging Effects of Stress Mediators. New England Journal of Medicine, 1998;338(3):171-177.

McEwen BS. Stress, adaptation, and disease. Allostasis and allostatic load. Ann NY Acad Sci. 1998; 840:33-44.

Perdrizet GA. Hans Selye and beyond: responses to stress. Cell Stress Chaperones. 1997 Dec;2(4):214-9.

Sajous, Charles E. de M. The Internal Secretions and the Practice of Medicine. Philadelphia, F. A. Davis Company, 1903. (10th ed., 1922).

Selye H. Forty years of stress research: principal remaining problems and misconceptions. Can Med Assoc. J. 1976 Jul 3;115(1):53-6.

Tattersall RB. Hypoadrenia or a "bit of Addison's Disease. Medical History. 1999;43:450-67.

CHAPTER TWO

Armario A. The hypothalamic-pituitary-adrenal axis: what can it tell us about stressors? CNS & Neuro Dis. 2006; 5:485+-501.

Davis EP, Glynn LM, Schetter CD, Hobel C, Chicz-Demet A, Sandman CA. Prenatal exposure to maternal depression and cortisol influences infant temperament. J. Am. Acad. Child Adolesc. Psychiatry. 2007;46(6):737-746.

The European Foundation for the Improvement of Living and Working Conditions. Wyattville Road, Loughlinstown, Dublin 18, Ireland. www.eurofound.europa.eu.

Gibbons C, Demptser M, Moutray, M. Stress and Eustress in Nursing Students. J Adv Nursing. 2008.61(3):282-90.

Kajantie E, Räikkönen K. Early life predictors of the physiological stress response later in life. Neurosci Biobehav Rev. 2010 Sep; 35 (1) :23-32.

Kajantie E, Phillips DI. The effects of sex and hormonal status on the physiological response to acute psychosocial stress. Psychoneuroendocrinology. 2006 Feb; 31 (2): 151-78.

Kajantie E. Fetal origins of stress-related adult disease. Ann N Y Acad Sci. 2006 Nov; 1083:11-27.

Kajantie E. Early-life events Effects on aging. Hormones (Athens). 2008 Apr-Jun; 7 (2): 101-13.

Kirschbaum C, Kudielka BM, Gaab J, Schommer NC, Hellhammer DH. Impact of gender, menstrual cycle phase, and oral contraceptives on the activity of the hypothalamus-pituitary-adrenal axis. Psychosom Med. 1999 Mar-Apr; 61 (2) :154-62.

Kudielka BM, Wust S. Human models in acute and chronic stress: assessing determinants of individual hypothalamus-pituitary-adrenal axis activity and reactivity. Stress. 2010;13(1):1-14.

Kudielka BM, Buske-Kirschbaum A, Hellhammer DH, Kirschbaum C. HPA axis responses to laboratory psychosocial stress in healthy elderly adults, younger adults, and children: impact of age and gender. Psychoneuroendocrinology. 2004 Jan; 29 (1) :83-98.

Kudielka BM, Schommer NC, Hellhammer DH, Kirschbaum C. Acute HPA axis responses, heart rate, and mood changes to psychosocial stress (TSST) in humans at different times of day. Psychoneuroendocrinology. 2004;(8) :983-92.

Meaney MJ, O'Donnell D, Rowe W, Tannenbaum B, Steverman A, Walker M, Nair NP, Lupien S. Individual differences in hypothalamic-pituitary-adrenal activity in later life and hippocampal aging. Exp Gerontol. 1995 May-Aug; 30 (3-4) :229-51.

Phillips DI. Programming of the stress response: a fundamental mechanism underlying the long-term effects of the fetal environment? J Intern Med. 2007 May; 261 (5) :453-60.

Veldhuis JD, Roelfsema F, Iranmanesh A, Carroll BJ, Keenan DM, Pincus SM. Basal, pulsatile, entropic (patterned), and spiky (staccato-like) properties of ACTH secretion: impact of age, gender, and body mass index. J Clin Endocrinol Metab. 2009 Oct; 94 (10) :4045-52.

CHAPTER THREE

Armario A. The hypothalamic-pituitary-adrenal axis: what can it tell us about stressors? CNS & Neuro Dis. 2006; 5:485-501.

Ahrentzen S. (1982) School Environments in Evans, G. (ed) Environmental stress pp. 224-255. Cambridge, NY: Cambridge University Press.

Chandola T, Heraclides A, Kumari M. Psychophysiological biomarkers of workplace stressors. Neurosci Biobehav Rev. 2010 Sep;35(1):51-7.

Eriksen, T. et al. The Scandinavian Way. Copenhagen Institute for Futures Studies. 2006.

Forbes.com http://www.forbes.com/2008/04/07/health-world-countries-forbeslife-cx_avd_0408health_slide_16.html?thisspeed=25000

Granger DA, Hibel LC, Fortunato CK, Kapelewski CH. Medication effects on salivary cortisol: Tactics and strategy to minimize impact in behavioral and developmental science. Psychoneuroendocrinology. 2009; 34:1437-1448.

Hibel LC, Granger DA, Kivlighan KT, Blair C, et al. Individual differences in salivary cortisol: Associations with common over-the-counter and prescription medication status in infants and their mothers. Hormones and Behavior. 2006; 50:293-300.

IMS Health, "IMS Health Reports U.S. Prescription Sales Grew 5.1 Percent in 2009, to $300.3 Billion" (April 1, 2010), online at http://www.imshealth.com.

Kaiser Family Foundation. Prescription Drug Trends. May 2010.

McEwen BS, Gianaros PJ. Central role of the brain in stress and adaptation: links to socioeconomic status, health, and disease. Ann NY Acad Sci. 2010; 1186:190-222.

Monica Higgins, Stacy E. McManus, Zibby Schwarzman. Work and Job Search Related Stress. Harvard Business Review. Publication date: Jul 07, 2004.

MedicineNet.com and the development of national registries for radiation; http://www.medterms.com/script/main/art.asp?articlekey=33284

National Sleep Foundation, 2005 Sleep in America pollNational Foundation of Brain Research (NIOSH) http://www.cdc.gov/niosh/topics/stress/

Rathus S, Nevid J. (2002) Psychology and the Challenges of Life: Adjustment in the New Millennium 8th edition. pp. 158 - 167. John Wiley & Sons.

Velickovic N, Djordjevic A, Matic G, Horvat A. Radiation-induced hyposuppression of the hypothalamic-pituitary-adrenal axis is associated with alterations of hippocampal corticosteroid receptor expression. Radiat Res. 2008 Apr;169(4):397-407.

Virgolini MB, Chen K, Weston DD, et al. Interactions of chronic lead exposure and intermittent stress: consequences for brain catecholamine systems and associated behaviours and HPA axis function. Toxicol Sci. 2005 Oct;87(2):469-82.

CHAPTER FOUR

ARK web site for Ortho-Molecular Products, "Is Adrenal Fatigue just a Phantom Internet Disease?" October 2010.

Armario A. The hypothalamic-pituitary-adrenal axis: what can it tell us about stressors? CNS Neurol Disord Drug Targets. 2006 Oct; 5(5): 485-501.

Baschetti R. "Chronic fatigue syndrome: a form of Addison's Disease." J Intern Med. 2000; 247:737-739.

Baschetti R. "Assessing chronic fatigue." QJM. 2003; 96(6):454.

Blakemore C, Jennett S. "Adrenal Glands." The Oxford Companion to the Body. 2001.

Beishuizen A, Thijs LG. Relative adrenal failure in intensive care: an identifiable problem requiring treatment? Best Prac Research Clin Endocrinol Metab. 2001; 15(4):513-531.

Chrousos G, Gold P. The concepts of stress and stress system disorders. JAMA. 1992; 267:1244-1252.

Doane LD, Adam EK. Loneliness and cortisol: momentary, day-to-day, and trait associations. Psychoneuroendocrinology. 2010 Apr;35(3):430-41.

Einaudi S, Matarazzo P, Peretta P, Grossetti R, et al. Hypothalamo-hypophysial dysfunction after traumatic brain injury in children and adolescents: a preliminary retrospective and prospective study. Journal of Pediatr Endocrinol Metab. 2006 May;19(5):691-703.

Freeman S. Biological Science. Prentice Hall; 2nd Pkg edition. 2004.

Heim C, Ehlert U, Hellhammer DH. The potential role of hypocortisolism in the pathophysiology of stress-related bodily disorders. Psychoneuroendocrinology. 2000; 25(1):1-35.

The Hormone Foundation (www.hormone.org).

Kajantie E, Räikkönen K. Early life predictors of the physiological stress response later in life. Neurosci Biobehav Rev. 2010 Sep; 35 (1) :23-32.

Keltikangas-Järvinen L, Räikkönen K, Hautanen A. Type A behavior and vital exhaustion as related to the metabolic hormonal variables of the hypothalamic-pituitary-adrenal axis. Behav Med. 1996 Spring;22(1):15-22.

Krahulik D, Zapletalova J, Frysak Z, Vaverka M. Dysfunction of hypothalamic-hypophysial axis after traumatic brain injury in adults. J Neurosurg. 2010;113(3):581-4.

Tintera JW. The hypoadrenocortical state and its management. New York State Journal of Medicine. 1955. v. 55; (13): 1869-76.

Van Voorhees E, Scarpa A. The effects of child maltreatment on the hypothalamic-pituitary-adrenal axis. Trauma Violence Abuse. 2004 Oct;5(4):333-52.

Wilson JL, Adrenal Fatigue, the 21st Century Syndrome. Smart Publications. Petaluma, CA 2001.

CHAPTER FIVE

Aardal-Eriksson E, Karlberg BE, Holm AC. Salivary cortisol--an alternative to serum cortisol determinations in dynamic function tests. Clin Chem Lab Med. 1998 Apr; 36 (4): 215-22.

LENA D. EDWARDS MD, FAARM

Arafah BM, Nishiyama FJ, Tlaygeh H, Hejal R. Measurement of salivary cortisol concentration in the assessment of adrenal function in critically ill subjects: A surrogate marker of the circulating free cortisol. J Clin Endocrinol Metab. 2007; 92: 2965–2971.

Bengtsson I, Lissner L, Ljung T, Rosengren A, Thelle D, Währborg P. The cortisol awakening response and the metabolic syndrome in a population-based sample of middle-aged men and women. Metabolism. 2010 Jul; 59 (7) :1012-9.

Cleare AJ, Miell J, Heap E, Sookdeo S, et al. Hypothalamo-pituitary-adrenal axis dysfunction in chronic fatigue syndrome, and the effects of low-dose hydrocortisone therapy. J Clin Endocrinol Metab. 2001 Aug;86(8):3545-54.

Clow A, Thorn L, Evans P, Hucklebridge F. The awakening cortisol response: methodological issues and significance. Stress. 2004 Mar; 7 (1) :29-37.

Cleare AJ et al. Urinary free cortisol in chronic fatigue syndrome. Am J Psychiatry. 2001; 158:641-3.

Gatti R, Antonelli G, Prearo M, Spinella P, Cappellin E, De Palo EF. Cortisol assays and diagnostic laboratory procedures in human biological fluids. Clin Biochem. 2009 Aug; 42 (12) :1205-17.

Gozansky WS, Lynn JS, Laudenslager ML, Kohrt WM. Salivary cortisol determined by enzyme immunoassay is preferable to serum total cortisol for assessment of dynamic hypothalamic--pituitary--adrenal axis activity. Clin Endocrinol (Oxf). 2005 Sep; 63 (3): 336-41.

Granger DA, Hibel LC, Fortunato CK, Kapelewski CH. Medication effects on salivary cortisol: Tactics and strategy to minimize impact in behavioral and developmental science. Psychoneuroendocrinology. 2009; 34:1437-1448.

Henry Wellcome Laboratories for Integrative Neuroscience and Endocrinology, University of Bristol, Bristol, UK. david.jessop@bris.ac.uk

Holtorf KH. Diagnosis and Treatment of Hypothalamic-Pituitary-Adrenal (HPA) Axis Dysfunction in Patients with Chronic Fatigue Syndrome (CFS) and Fibromyalgia (FM). J Chr Fatigue Syn. 2008; 14(3):1-14.

Jessop DS, Turner-Cobb JM., Measurement and meaning of salivary cortisol: a focus on health and disease in children. Stress. 2008;11(1):1-14. Epub 2007 Jul 16.

Kirschbaum, Kudielka, Gaab, et al. Impact of Gender, menstrual cycle phase, and oral contraceptives on the activity of the hypothalamus-pituitary-adrenal axis. Psychosom. Med. 1999;61:154-162.

Kirschbaum, Scherer, Strasburger. Pituitary and adrenal hormone responses to pharmacological, physical, and psychological stimulation in habitual smokers and nonsmokers. Clin Invest. 1994;72:804-810.

Kudielka, et al. Why do we respond so differently? Reviewing determinants of human salivary cortisol responses to challenge. Psychoneuroendocrinology. 2009; 34:2-18.

Lovallo, Farag, Vincent, et al. Cortisol responses to mental stress, exercise, and meals following caffeine intake in men and women. Pharmacol Biochem Behav. 2006;83:441-7.

Nieman L, Biller B, Findling J, Newell-Price J, Savage M et al. The Diagnosis of Cushing's Syndrome: An Endocrine Society Clinical Practice Guideline. First published in the Journal of Clinical Endocrinology & Metabolism, May 2008, 93(5): 1526–1540.

Persson R, Garde AH, Hansen AM, Osterberg K, Larsson B, Orbaek P, Karlson B. Seasonal variation in human salivary cortisol concentration. Chronobiol Int. 2008 Nov; 25 (6) :923-37.

Poll E, Kreitschmann-Andermahr I, Langejuergen Y, et al. Saliva collection method affects predictability of serum cortisol. Clinica Chimica Acta. 2007; 382:15–19.

Schwartz ET, Holtorf K. Hormones in wellness and disease prevention: common practices, current state of the evidence, and questions for the future. Primary Care. 2008 Dec;35(4):669-705.

Smith AP. Stress, breakfast cereal consumption, and cortisol. Nutr Neurosci. 2002;5:141-4.

Smyth JM, Ockenfels MC, Gorin AA, et al. Individual differences in the diurnal cycle of cortisol. Psychoneuroendocrinol. 1997;22:89-105.

Stone AA, Schwartz JE, Smyth J, et al. Individual differences in the diurnal cycle of salivary free cortisol: a replication of flattened cycles for some individuals. Psychoneuroendocrinol. 2001;26:295-306.

Törnhage CJ. Salivary cortisol for assessment of hypothalamic-pituitary-adrenal axis function. Neuroimmunomodulation. 2009; 16 (5) :284-9.

Vining RF, McGinley RA, Maksvytis JJ, Ho KY. Salivary cortisol: a better measure of adrenal cortical function than serum cortisol. Ann Clin Biochem. 1983 Nov; 20 (Pt 6):329-35.

CHAPTER SIX

Akishita M, Hashimoto M, Ohike Y, Ogawa S, et al. Low testosterone level as a predictor of cardiovascular events in Japanese men with coronary risk factors. Atherosclerosis. 2010 May;210(1):232-6.

Akishita M, Hashimoto M, Ohike Y, Ogawa S, Iijima K, Eto M, Ouchi Y. Low testosterone level is an independent determinant of endothelial dysfunction in men. Hypertens Res. 2007 Nov; 30(11):1029-34.

Berga SL, Loucks TL. The diagnosis and treatment of stress-induced anovulation. Minerva Ginecol. 2005 Feb;57(1):45-54.

LENA D. EDWARDS MD, FAARM

Cagnacci A, Cannoletta M, Caretto S, Zanin R, et al. Increased cortisol level: a possible link between climacteric symptoms and cardiovascular risk factors. Menopause. 2011 Mar;18(3):273-8.

Campino C, Valenzuela F, Arteaga E, et al. Melatonin reduces cortisol response to ACTH in humans. Rev Med Chil. 2008 Nov;136(11):1390-7.

Chrousos GP, Torpy DJ, Gold PW. Interactions between the hypothalamic-pituitary-adrenal axis and the female reproductive system: clinical implications. Ann Intern Med. 1998 Aug 1;129(3):229-40.

Clemmons DR. The diagnosis and treatment of growth hormone deficiency in adults. Curr Opinion Endocrinology. Diabetes and Obesity. 2010; 17(4): 377–383.

Helmreich DL, Parfitt DB, Lu XY, Akil H, Watson SJ. Relation between the hypothalamic-pituitary-thyroid (HPT) axis and the hypothalamic-pituitary-adrenal (HPA) axis during repeated stress. Neuroendocrinology. 2005;81(3):183-92.

Kim C, et al. Effect of hormone replacement therapy on lipoprotein. Arch Intern Med. 1996;156:1693-1700.

L'hermite M, Simoncini T, Fuller S, Genazzani , AR. Maturitas. Could transdermal estradiol + progesterone be a safer postmenopausal HRT? 2008 Jul-Aug;60(3-4): 185-201. Epub 2008 Sep 5.

Magiakou, MA, Mastorakos, G, Webster E, Chrousos GP. The Hypothalamic-Pituitary-Adrenal Axis and the Female Reproductive System. Ann N Y Acad Sci. 1997 Jun 17;816:42-56.

Pal L, Bevilacqua K, Santoro NF. Chronic psychosocial stressors are detrimental to ovarian reserve: a study of infertile women. J Psychosom Obstet Gynaecol. 2010 Sep;31(3):130-9.

Popma A, et al. Cortisol moderates the relationship between testosterone and aggression in delinquent male adolescents. Biol Psychiatry. 2007 Feb 1;61(3):405-11.

Reddy DS. Neurosteroids: endogenous role in the human brain and therapeutic potentials. Prog Brain Res. 2010;186:113-37.

Rios ERV, Venancio, ET, Rocha NFM et al. Melatonin: Pharmacological Aspects and Clinical Trends. Int J Neuroscience. 2010;120:583-590.

Stein DG, Wright DW. Progesterone in the clinical treatment of acute traumatic brain injury. Expert Opin Investig Drugs. 2010 Jul;19(7):847-57.

Taskinen MR, Puolakka J, Pyörälä T, Luotola H, et al. Hormone replacement therapy lowers plasma Lp(a) concentrations. Comparison of cyclic transdermal and continuous estrogen-progestin regimens. Arterioscler Thromb Vasc Biol. 1996 Oct;16(10):1215-21.

Terburg D, Morgan B, van Honk J, The testosterone-cortisol ratio: A hormonal marker for proneness to social aggression. Int J Law Psychiatry. 2009 Jul-Aug;32(4):216-23.

Torner L, Neumann ID. The brain prolactin system: involvement in stress response adaptations in lactation. Stress. 2002 Dec;5(4):249-57.

Traish AM, Saad F, Feeley RJ, Guay A. The dark side of testosterone deficiency: III. Cardiovascular disease. J Androl. 2009 Sep-Oct;30(5):477-94.

Van Bokhoven I, et al. Salivary testosterone and aggression, delinquency, and social dominance in a population-based longitudinal study of adolescent males. Horm Behav. 2006 Jun;50(1):118-25.

Woods NF, Carr MC, Tao EY, Taylor HJ, Mitchell ES. Increased urinary cortisol levels during the menopausal transition. Menopause. 2006 Mar-Apr;13(2):212-21.

Xiao G, Wei J, Yan W, Wang W, Lu Z. Improved outcomes from the administration of progesterone for patients with acute severe traumatic brain injury: a randomized controlled trial. Crit Care. 2008;12(2):R61.

CHAPTER SEVEN

Aboa-Eboulé C, Brisson C, Maunsell E, Mâsse B, Bourbonnais R, et al. Job strain and risk of acute recurrent coronary heart disease events. JAMA. 2007 Oct 10;298(14):1652-60.

al'Absi M, Arnett DK. Adrenocortical responses to psychological stress and risk for hypertension. Biomed Pharmacother. 2000 Jun;54(5):234-44.

Anagnostis P, Vasilios GA, Tziomalos K, Karagiannis A, Mikhailidis DP. The pathogenetic role of cortisol in the metabolic syndrome: a hypothesis. J Clin Endocrinol Metab. 2009;94:2692-2701.

Analava Mitra, Diabetes and Stress: A Review. Ethno-Med. 2(2): 131-135, 2008.

Arnaldi G, Scandali VM, Trementino L, Cardinaletti M, Appolloni G, Boscaro M. Pathophysiology of dyslipidemia in Cushing's syndrome. Neuroendocrinology. 2010; 92 Suppl 1:86-90.

Baltrusch HJ, Stangel W, Titze I. Stress, cancer and immunity. New developments in biopsychosocial and psychoneuroimmunologic research. Acta Neurol (Napoli). 1991 Aug;13(4):315-27.

Basta M, Chrousos GP, Vela-Bueno A, Vgontzas AN. Chronic insomnia and the stress system. Sleep Med Clin. 2007; 2 (2) :279-291.

Batemen A, Singh A, Kral T, Solomon S. The immune-hypothalamic-pituitary-adrenal axis. Endocrinol Rev. 1989;10:92-112.

Benedict C, Kern W, Schmid SM, Schultes B, et al. Early morning rise in hypothalamic-pituitary-adrenal activity: a role for maintaining the brain's energy balance. Psychoneuroendocrinology. 2009 Apr; 34 (3) :455-62.

Bonnet F, Irving K, Terra JL, Nony P, Berthezène F, Moulin P. Anxiety and depression are associated with unhealthy lifestyle in patients at risk of cardiovascular disease. Atherosclerosis. 2005;178(2):339-344.

Bosma H, Marmot MG, Hemingway H, Nicholson AC, Brunner E, Stansfeld SA.Low job control and risk of coronary heart disease in Whitehall II (prospective cohort) study. BMJ. 1997 Feb 22;314(7080):558-65.

Buckley TM, Schatzberg AF. On the interactions of the hypothalamic-pituitary-adrenal (HPA) axis and sleep: normal HPA axis activity and circadian rhythm, exemplary sleep disorders. J Clin Endocrinol Metab. 2005 May;90(5):3106-14.

Carmen Wong KY, Wong V, Ho JT, et al. High cortisol levels in hyperglycaemic myocardial infarct patients signify stress hyperglycaemia and predict subsequent normalization of glucose tolerance. Clin Endocrinol (Oxf). 2010; 72 (2) :189-95.

Carroll BJ, Cassidy F, Naftolowitz D, Tatham NE, et al. Pathophysiology of hypercortisolism in depression. Acta Psychiatr Scand Suppl. Acta Psychiatr Scand Suppl. 2007;(433):90-103.

Chanson P, Salenave S. Metabolic syndrome in Cushing's syndrome. Neuroendocrinology. 2010; 92 Suppl 1:96-101.

Chiodini I, Mascia ML, Muscarella S, Battista C, Minisola S, et al. Subclinical hypercortisolism among outpatients referred for osteoporosis. Ann Intern Med. 2007 Oct 16;147(8):541-8.

Chiodini I, Scillitani A. Role of cortisol hypersecretion in the pathogenesis of osteoporosis. Recenti Prog Med. 2008 Jun;99(6):309-13.

Chrousos GP. The role of stress and the hypothalamic-pituitary-adrneal axis in the pathogenesis of the metabolic syndrome: neuroendocrine and target tissue-related causes. Int J Obes Relat Metab Disord. 2000; 24:S50-55.

Chrousos GP, Gold PW. The concepts of stress and stress system disorders: overview of physical and behavioral homeostasis. JAMA. 1992;267:1244-125.

Colao A. The GH-IGF-I axis and the cardiovascular system: clinical implications. Clin Endocrinol (Oxf). 2008 Sep; 69 (3) :347-58.

Csernansky JG, Dong H, Fagan AM, Wang L, Xiong C, Holtzman DM, Morris JC. Plasma cortisol and progression of dementia in subjects with Alzheimer-type dementia. Am J Psychiatry. 2006;163:2164–2.

Cummings SR, Melton LJ. Epidemiology and outcomes of osteoporotic fractures. Lancet 2002;359:1761.

Dallman M, Pecoraro N, Akana S, et al. Chronic stress and obesity: A new view of comfort food. PNAS. 2003;100:11696-701.

Davis KL, Davis BM, Greenwald BS, Mohs RC, Mathé AA, Johns CA, Horvath TB. Cortisol and Alzheimer's disease, I: Basal studies. Am J Psychiatry. 1986;143:300–305169.

Dinan TG, Quigley EM, Ahmed SM, Scully P, O'Brien S, O'Mahony L, O'Mahony S, Shanahan F, Keeling PW. Hypothalamic-pituitary-gut axis dysregulation in irritable bowel syndrome: plasma cytokines as a potential biomarker? Gastroenterology. 2006 Feb;130(2):304-11.

Donoho CJ, Weigensberg MJ, Emken BA, Hsu JW, Spruijt-Metz D. Stress and abdominal fat: preliminary evidence of moderation by the cortisol awakening response in hispanic peripubertal girls. Obesity (Silver Spring). 2010 Dec 2 [Epub ahead of print].

Drossman DA. Abuse, trauma, and GI illness: is there a link?. Am J Gastroenterol. 2011 Jan;106(1):14-25.

Effo N. Who are candidates for prevention and treatment for osteoporosis? Osteoporosis Int. 1997;7:1.

Elenkov IJ, Chrousos GP. Stress hormones, Th1/Th2 patters, pro/anti-inflammatory cytokines and susceptibility to disease. Trends Endocrinol Metab. 1999;10:359.

Epel ES, McEwen B, Seeman T, Matthews K, Castellazzo G, Brownell KD, Bell J, Ickovics JR. Stress and body shape: stress-induced cortisol secretion is consistently greater among women with central fat. Psychosom Med. 2000 Sep-Oct;62(5):623-32.

Epel S. Psychological and metabolic stress: A recipe for accelerated cellular aging? Hormones. 2009;8:7-22.

Felšöci M, Schroner Z, Petrovicová J, Lazúrová I. Relationship between type 2 diabetes mellitus and hypothalamic-pituitary-adrenal axis. Wien Klin Wochenschr. 2011 Jan;123 (1-2):28-33.

Gold PW, Chrousos GP. Organization of the stress system and its dysregulation in melancholic and atypical depression: high vs low CRH/NE states. Mol Psychiatry. 2002; 7(3):254-75.

Gullberg B, Johnell O, Kanis JA (1997) World-wide projections for hip fracture. Osteoporos Int.7:407.

Habib KE, Weld KP, Rice KC, Pushkas J, et al. Oral administration of a corticotrophin-releasing hormone receptor antagonist significantly attenuates behavioral, neuroendocrine, and autonomic responses to stress in primates. Proc Natl Acad Sci USA. 2000. May 23;97(11):6079-84.

Irie M, Asami S, Nagata S, Miyata M, Kasai H. Relationships between perceived workload, stress and oxidative DNA damage. Int Arch Occup Environ Health. 2001 Mar;74(2):153-7.

Johnson EO, Kamilaris TC, Chrousos GP, Gold PW. Mechanisms of Stress: A dynamic overview of hormonal and behavioral homeostasis. Neurosc Behav Rev. 1992;16:115-130.

Kaltsas G, Makras P. Skeletal diseases in Cushing's syndrome: osteoporosis versus arthropathy. Neuroendocrinology. 2010;92 Suppl 1:60-4.

Kimonides VG, Khatibi NH, Svendsen CN, Sofroniew MV, Herbert J. Dehydroepiandrosterone (DHEA) and DHEA-sulfate (DHEAS) protect hippocampal neurons against excitatory amino acid-induced neurotoxicity. Proc Natl Acad Sci USA. 1998;95:1852-1857.

Kimonides VG, Spillantini MG, Sofroniew MV, Fawcett JW, Herbert J. Dehydroepiandrosterone antagonizes the neurotoxic effects of corticosterone and translocation of stress-activated protein kinase 3 in hippocampal primary cultures. Neuroscience. 1999;89:429-436.

Kuper H, Marmot M. Job strain, job demands, decision latitude, and risk of coronary heart disease within the Whitehall II study. J Epidemiol Community Health. 2003 Feb;57(2):147-53.

Kyrou I, Chrousos GP, Tsigos C. Stress, visceral obesity, and metabolic complications. Ann N Y Acad Sci. 2006 Nov;1083:77-110.

Kyrou I, Tsigos C. Stress hormones: physiological stress and regulation of metabolism. Curr Opin Pharmacol. 2009 Dec;9(6):787-93.

Kyrou I, Tsigos C. Chronic stress, visceral obesity and gonadal dysfunction. Hormones (Athens). 2008 Oct-Dec;7(4):287-93.

Lanfumey L, Mongeau R, Cohen-Salmon C, Hamon M. Corticosteroid-serotonin interactions in the neurobiological mechanisms of stress-related disorders. Neurosci Biobehav Rev. 2008 Aug;32(6):1174-84.

Lerebours E, Gower-Rousseau C, Merle V, Brazier F, et al. Stressful life events as a risk factor for inflammatory bowel disease onset: A population-based case-control study. Am J Gastroenterol. 2007 Jan;102(1):122-31.

Lissoni P, Brivio F, Fumagalli L, Messina G, et al. Immune and endocrine mechanisms of advanced cancer-related hypercortisolemia. In Vivo. 2007 Jul-Aug;21(4):647-50.

Lupien SJ, de Leon M, de Santi S, Convit A, Tarshish C, Nair NP, Thakur M, McEwen BS, Hauger RL, Meaney MJ. Cortisol levels during human aging predict hippocampal atrophy and memory deficits. Nat Neurosci. 1998 May;1(1): 69-73.

Mawdsley JE, Rampton DS. Psychological stress in IBD: new insights into pathogenic and therapeutic implications. Gut. 2005 Oct; 54(10):1481-91.

McEwen BS. Sleep deprivation as a neurobiologic and physiologic stressor: Allostasis and allostatic load. Metabolism. 2006 Oct; 55 (10 Suppl 2):S20-3.

McEwen BS. Protective and damaging effects of stress mediators: central role of the brain. Dialogues Clin Neurosci. 2006;8(4):367-81.

McEwen BS. Physiology and neurobiology of stress and adaptation: central role of the brain. Physiol Rev. 2007 Jul; 87(3):873-904.

McEwen BS. Central effects of stress hormones in health and disease: understanding the protective and damaging effects of stress and stress mediators. Eur J Pharm. 2008;583:174-185.

McEwen BS. Possible mechanisms for atrophy of the human hippocampus. Mol Psychiatry. 1997;2:255-262.

Moreno-Smith M, Lutgendorf SK, Sood AK. Impact of stress on cancer metastasis. Future Oncol. 2010 Dec;6(12):1863-81.

Morin, Charles M. (2003). Insomnia. New York: Kluwer Academic/Plenum Publ. p. 28.

Moyer AE, Rodin J, Grilo CM, Cummings N, Larson LM, Rebuffé-Scrive M. Stress-induced cortisol response and fat distribution in women. Obes Res. 1994 May;2(3):255-62.

National Institute of Mental Health. Prevalence of Serious Mental Illness Among U.S. Adults by Age, Sex, and Race. http://www.nimh.nih.gov/statistics/SMI_AASR.shtml

Palmieri VO, Grattagliano I, Portincasa P, Palasciano G. Systemic oxidative alterations are associated with visceral adiposity and liver steatosis in patients with metabolic syndrome. J Nutr. 2006;136:3022-26.

Pariante CM, Thomas SA, Lovestone S, Makoff A, Kerwin RW. Do antidepressants regulate how cortisol affects the brain? Psychoneuroendocrinology. 2004 May;29(4):423-47.

Peeke PM, Chrousos GP. Hypercortisolism and obesity. Ann N Y Acad Sci. 1995 Dec 29; 771:665-76.

Pou KM, Massaro JM, Hoffman U, et al. Visceral and subcutaneous adipose tissue volumes are cross-sectionally related to markers of inflammation and oxidative stress: the Framingham Heart Study. Circulation. 2007:1234-41.

Pouwer F, Kupper N, Adriaanse MC. Does emotional stress cause type 2 diabetes mellitus? A review from the European depression in diabetes (EDID) research consortium. Discov Med. 2010 Feb;9(45):112-8.

Rabin DS, Gold PW, Margioris AN, Chrousos GP. Stress and reproduction: Physiological interactions between the stress and reproductive axes. In: Chrousos GP, Loriau DL,

Gold PW, eds. Mechanisms of physical and emotional stress. Vol 245. Advances in experimental medicine and biology. New York: Prentice Hall; 1988:377-387.

Räikkönen K, Lassila R, Keltikangas-Järvinen L, Hautanen A. Association of chronic stress with plasminogen activator inhibitor-1 in healthy middle-aged men. Arterioscler Thromb Vasc Biol. 1996 Mar;16(3):363-7.

Räikkönen K, Hautanen A, Keltikangas-Järvinen L. Feelings of exhaustion, emotional distress, and pituitary and adrenocortical hormones in borderline hypertension. J Hypertens. 1996 Jun;14(6):713-8.

Rebuffé-Scrive M, Walsh UA, McEwen B, Rodin J. Effect of chronic stress and exogenous glucocorticoids on regional fat distribution and metabolism. Physiol Behav. 1992 Sep;52(3):583-90.

Rod NH, Grønbaek M, Schnohr P, Prescott E, Kristensen TS. Perceived stress as a risk factor for changes in health behaviour and cardiac risk profile: a longitudinal study. J Intern Med. 2009;266(5):467-475.

Santos J, Alonso C, Vicario M, Ramos L, Lobo B, Malagelada JR. Neuropharmacology of stress-induced mucosal inflammation: implications for inflammatory bowel disease and irritable bowel syndrome. Curr Mol Med. 2008 Jun;8(4):258-73.

Sapolsky RM. Why stress is bad for your brain. Science. 1996 Aug 9;273(5276):749-50.

Sapolsky RM. Glucocorticoids and hippocampal atrophy in neuropsychiatric disorders. Arch Gen Psychiatry. 2000 Oct;57(10):925-35.

Saruta T. Mechanism of glucocorticoid-induced hypertension. Hypertens Res. 1996 Mar;19(1):1-8.

Sheline YI, Sanghavi M, Mintun MA, Gado MH. Depression duration but not age predicts hippocampal volume loss in medically healthy women with recurrent major depression. J Neurosci. 1999 Jun 15;19(12):5034-43.

Smith GD, Ben-Shlomo Y, Beswick A, Yarnell J, Lightman S, Elwood P. Cortisol, testosterone, and coronary heart disease: prospective evidence from the Caerphilly study. Circulation. 2005 Jul 19;112(3):332-40.

Smith MA, Kling MA, Whitfield HJ, Brandt HA, Demitrack MA, Geracioti TD, Chrousos GP, Gold PW. Corticotropin-releasing hormone: from endocrinology to psychobiology. Horm Res. 1989;31(1-2):66-71.

Stansfeld SA, Fuhrer R, Shipley MJ, Marmot MG. Psychological distress as a risk factor for coronary heart disease in the Whitehall II Study. Int J Epidemiol. 2002 Feb;31(1):248-55.

Surwit RS, van Tilburg MA, Zucker N, McCaskill CC, Parekh P, Feinglos MN, Edwards CL, Williams P, Lane JD. Stress management improves long-term glycemic control in type 2 diabetes. Diabetes Care. 2002 Jan;25 (1):30-4.

Tenerz A, Nilsson G, Forberg R, Ohrvik J, Malmberg K, Berne C, Leppert J. Basal glucometabolic status has an impact on long-term prognosis following an acute myocardial infarction in non-diabetic patients. J Intern Med. 2003 Nov; 254 (5) :494-503.

Toussaint O, Michiels C, Raes M, Remacle J. Cellular aging and the importance of energetic factors. Exp Gerontol. 1995;30:1-22.

Tsigos C, Chrousos GP. Hypothalamic-pituitary-adrenal axis, neuroendocrine factors and stress. Psychosom Res. 2002; 53(4):865-71.

Vgontzas AN, Mastorakos G, Bixler EO, Kales A, Gold PW, Chrousos GP. Sleep deprivation effects on the activity of the hypothalamic-pituitary-adrenal and growth axes: potential clinical implications. Clin Endocrinol (Oxf). 1999 Aug; 51(2):205-15.

Vgontzas AN, Chrousos GP. Sleep, the hypothalamic-pituitary-adrenal axis, and cytokines: multiple interactions and disturbances in sleep disorders. Endocrinol Metab Clin North Am. 2002 Mar; 31(1):15-36.

Vogelzangs N, Beekman AT, Milaneschi Y, Bandinelli S, Ferrucci L, Penninx BW. Urinary cortisol and six-year risk of all-cause and cardiovascular mortality. J Clin Endocrinol Metab. 2010 Nov; 95 (11):4959-64.

Webster Marketon JI, Glaser R. Stress hormones and immune function. Cell Immunol. 2008 Mar-Apr;252(1-2):16-26.

Whitworth JA, Williamson PM, Mangos G, Kelly JJ. Cardiovascular consequences of cortisol excess. Vasc Health Risk Manag. 2005;1(4):291-9.

Willis T. Pharmaceutice rationalis sive diatriba de medicamentorum operationibus in humano corpore. [Oxford]: E Theatro Sheldoniano, M.DC.LXXV, 1675.

U.S. Obesity Trends: Trends by State 1985–2009. The incidence of obesity in the U.S. has doubled in the last decade (Center for Disease Control) http://www.cdc.gov/obesity/data/trends.html

CHAPTER EIGHT

Adams EK, Gunnar MR. Relationship functioning and home and work demands predict individual differences in the diurnal cycle of cortisol in women Psychneuroendocrinology. 2001;26:189-208.

Abercombrie H. et. Al. Flattened cortisol rhythms in metastatic breast cancer patients. Psychoneuroendocrinology. 2004;29;1082–1092.

Ball TM, Anderson D, Minto J, Halonen M. Cortisol circadian rhythms and stress responses in infants at risk of allergic disease. Amer Acad Allergy. 2006;117:306-311. Baschetti R. Chronic fatigue. CMAJ. 2006 Aug 15;175(4):386.

Baschetti R. Chronic fatigue syndrome: a form of Addison's Disease. J Intern Med. 2000; 247:737-739.

Baschetti R. Chronic fatigue syndrome, exercise, cortisol and lymphadenopathy. J Intern Med. 2005 Sep;258(3):291-2.

Behan, WM. Muscles, Mitochondria and Myalgia. J. Pathology 1992;166:213-14.

Behen, WH, More, IR, Behan, PO. Mitochondrial abnormalities in postviral fatigue syndrome. Acta Neuropathol 1991;83:61-65.

Berg D, Berg LH, Couvaras J. Is CFS/FM due to an undefined hypercoaguable state brought on by immune activation of coagulation. Does adding anticoagulant therapy improve CFS/FM patient symptoms? AACFS Proceedings, Cambridge, MA. October1998;62:10-12.

Bilginer Y, Topaloglu R, Alikasifoglu A, Kara N, Besbas N, et al. Low cortisol levels in active juvenile idiopathic arthritis. Clin Rheumatol. 2010;29:309-314.

Blackburn-Munro G, Blackburn-Munro R. Pain in the brain: are hormones to blame? Trends Endocrinol Metab. 2003 Jan;14(1):20-7.

Bower JE, et al. Inflammatory responses to psychological stress in fatigued breast cancer survivors: relationship to glucocorticoids. Brain, Behavior, and Immunity. 2007; 21:251–258.

Cash JM, Crofford LJ, Gallucci WT, Sternberg EM, Gold PW, Chrousos GP, Wilder RL. Pituitary-adrenal axis responsiveness to ovine corticotropin releasing hormone in patients with rheumatoid arthritis treated with low dose prednisone. J Rheumatol. 1992 Nov;19(11):1692-6.

Chrousos, GP. Stress, chronic inflammation, and emotional and physical wellbeing: concurrent effects and chronic sequelae. J Allergy Clin Immunol. 2000;106:275–91.

Chrousos GP, Gold PW. The concept of stress and stress system disorders. Overview of physical and behavioural homeostasis. J Am Med Dir Assoc. 1992;267:1244–52.

Cleare AJ, Miell J, Heap E, Sookdeo S, et al. Hypothalamic-pituitary-adrenal axis dysfunction in chronic fatigue syndrome and the effects of low-dose hydrocortisone therapy. J Clin Endocrinol Metab. 2001;86(8):3545-3554.

Delahanty DL, Dougall AL, Craig KJ, Jemkins FJ, Baum A. Chronic stress and natural killer cell activity after exposure to traumatic death. Psychosom Med. 1997;59:467-76.

Delahanty DL, Raimonde AJ, Spoonster E, et al. Injury severity, prior trauma history, urinary cortisol levels, and acute PTSD in motor vehicle accident victims. J Anx Disord 2003;17:149–164.

Demitrack MA, Dale JK, Straus SE, Laue L, Listwak SJ, Kruesi MJ, Chrousos GP, Gold PW. Evidence for impaired activation of the hypothalamic-pituitary-adrenal axis in patients with chronic fatigue syndrome. J Clin Endocrinol Metab. 1991;73(6):1224-34.

Elenkov & Chrousos. Stress Hormones, Th1/Th2 patterns, Pro/Anti-inflammatory Cytokines and Susceptibility to Disease. Trends Endocrinol Metab. 1999;10:359-368.

Englebienne P, Verhas M, Herst CV, Ke Meirleir K. Type I interferons induce proteins susceptible to act as thyroid receptor (TR) corepressors and to signal the TR for destruction by the proteasome: possible etiology for unexplained chronic fatigue. Med Hypoth 2003;60(2):175-180.

Elwan O, Mohamed Abdella M, El Bayad AB, Hamdy S. Hormonal changes in headache patients. J Neurol Sci. 1991;106:75–81.

Fletcher MA, Maher, KJ, Klimas, NG. Natural killer cell function in chronic fatigue syndrome. Clinical and Applied Immunology Reviews. 2002;2(2):129-139.

FMAware.org: http://www.fmaware.org/site/PageServera6cc.html?pagename=fibromyalgia_affected

Fries E, Dettenborn L, Kirschbaum C. The cortisol awakening response (CAR): facts and future directions. Int J Psychophysiol. 2009 Apr;72(1):67-73.

Fries E, Hesse J, Hellhammer J, Hellhammer DH. A new view on hypocortisolism. Psychoneuroendocrinology. 2005;10:1010-6.

Galli U, Gaab J, Ettlin DA, Ruggia F, Ehlert U, Palla S. Enhanced negative feedback sensitivity of the hypothalamus–pituitary–adrenal axis in chronic myogenous facial pain. Eur J Pain 2009;13:600–5.

Gold PW, Chrousos GP. Organization of the stress system and its dysregulation in melancholic and atypical depression: high vs low CRH/NE states. Mol Psychiatry. 2002; 7:254-275.

Griep RA, van Twisk C, van Beckhoven JR, van der Wolf JM, Schots A. Development of specific recombinant monoclonal antibodies against the lipopolysaccharide of ralstonia solanacearum race 3. Phytopathology. 1998 Aug;88(8):795-803.

Gunnar MR, Vazquez DM. Low cortisol and a flattening of expected daytime rhythm: Potential indices of risk in human development. Dev Psychopathology. 2001;13:515-538.

Gur A, Cevik R, Sarac J, Colpan L, et al. Hypothalamic-pituitary-gonadal axis and cortisol in young women with primary fibromyalgia: the potential roles of depression, fatigue, and sleep disturbance in the occurrence of hypocortisolism. Ann Rheum Dis. 2004;63:1504-1506.

Hart BL. Biological basis of the behavior os sick animals. Neurosci Biobehav Rev. 1988;12:123-137.

Heim C, Ehlert U, Hanker JP, Hallhammer DH. Abuse-related posttraumatic stress disorder and alterations of the hypothalamic-pituitary-adrenal axis in women with chronic pelvic pain. Psychosom Med. 1998;60:309-318.

Heim C, Ehlert U, Hellhammer DH. The potential role of hypocortisolism in the pathphysiology of stress-related bodily disorders. Psychoneuroendocrinology. 2000;25:1-35.

Holtorf, K. Diagnosis and treatment of hypothalamic-pituitary-adrenal (hpa) axis dysfunctionin patients with chronic fatigue syndrome (CFS) and fibromyalgia (FM). J Chr Fatigue Syn. 2008; 14(3):1-14.

Jo Nijs J et al. High prevalence of Mycoplasma infections among European chronic fatigue syndrome patients. Examination of four Mycoplasma species in blood of chronic fatigue syndrome patients. FEMS Immunology & Medical Microbiology 2002;34:209-214.

Klimas NG et al. Immunologic abnormalities in chronic fatigue syndrome. J Clin Microbiology. 1990;28(6):1403-1410.

Kivimaki M, Leino-Arjas P, Virtanen M, Elovainio M, Keltikangas-Jarvinen L, et al. Work stress and incidence of newly-diagnosed fibromyalgia: prospective cohort study. J Psychosom Res. 2004 Nov;57(5):415-6.

Lampe A, Doering S, Rumpold G, Solder E, Krismer M, Kantner-Rumplmair W, Schubert C, Sollner W. Chronic pain syndromes and their relation to childhood abuse and stressful life events. J. Psychosom Res 2003;54, 361–367.

Lévi F, Focan C, Karaboué A, de la Valette V, Focan-Henrard D, Baron B, Kreutz F, Giacchetti S. Implications of circadian clocks for the rhythmic delivery of cancer therapeutics. Adv Drug Deliv Rev. 2007 Aug 31;59(9-10):1015-35.

Marik PE, Pastores SM, Annane D, et al. Recommendations for the diagnosis and management of corticosteroid insufficiency in critically ill adult patients: consensus statements from an international task force by the American College of Crit Care Med 2008;36:1937–1949.

Marik PE. Critical Illness-related corticosteroid insufficiency. Chest. 2009;135:181–193.

Masi AT, Chatterton RT, Aldag JC. Perturbations of hypothalamic-pituitary-gonadal axis and adrenal androgen functions in rheumatoid arthritis: an odyssey of hormonal relationships to the disease. Ann N Y Acad Sci. 1999 Jun 22;876:53-62.

Matthews K, Schwartz J, Cohen S, Seeman T. Diurnal cortisol decline is related to coronary calcification: CARDIA Study. Psychosomatic Med. 2006:68;657-661.

McFarlane AC, Atchison M, Yehuda R. The acute stress response following motor vehicle accidents and its relation to PTSD. Ann New York Acad Sci. 1997;821:437–441.

Metzger et al. Basal and suppressed salivary cortisol in female Vietnam nurse veterans with and without PTSD. Psychiatry Res. 2008;161:330-335.

Moldofsky H. Sleep and musculoskeletal pain. Am J Med. 1986;81:85-9.

Moldofsky H. Sleep and fibrositis syndrome. Rheum Dis Clin North Am. 1989;15:91-103.

Nater, et al. Trier Social Stress Test; Psychoneuroendocrinology. 2007;32:758-763.

Nicolson NA, van Diest R. Salivary cortisol patterns in vital exhaustion. J Psychosomatic Res. 2000;49:335-342.

Novartis Found Symp. 2000;227:119-36; discussion 136-42.

Peterson, A. L. Komaroff, and J. Ritz. Phenotypic and functional deficiency of natural killer cells in patients with chronic fatigue syndrome. J. Immunol. 1987;139:3306-3313.

Petrelluzzi KF, Garcia MC, Petta CA, Grassi-Kassisse DM, Spadari-Bratfisch RC. Salivary cortisol concentrations, stress and quality of life in women with endometriosis and chronic pelvic pain. Stress. 2008;11(5):390-7.

Pruessner JC, Hellhammer DH, Kirschbaum C. Burnout, perceived stress and salivary cortisol upon awakening. Psychosomatic Med. 1999;61:197-294.

Raison CL, Miller AH. When not enough is too much: the role of insufficient glucocorticoid signaling in the pathophysiology of stress-related disorders. Am J Psychiatry. 2003;160:1554-1565.

Reeves WC, Jones JF, Maloney E, Heim C, Hoaglin DC, Boneva RS, Morrisse M, Devlin R. Prevalence of chronic fatigue syndrome in metropolitan, urban, and rural Georgia. Popul Health Metr. 2007;5:5.

Riley MS, O'Brien CJ, McCluskey DR et al. Aerobic work capacity in patients with chronic fatigue syndrome. Brit Med J. 1990;301:953-6.

Rohleder N, Joksimovic L, Wolf JM, Kirschbaum C. Hypocortisolism and increased glucocorticoid sensitivity of pro-inflammatory cytokine production in Bosnian War refugees with Posttraumatic Stress Disorder. Bil Psych. 2004;55:745-751.

Rosmond R, Dallman M., Bjorntorp P. Stress related cortisol secretion in men: Relationships with abdominal obesity and endocrine, metabolic, and hemodynamic abnormalities. J Clin Endocrinol Metab. 1998:83;1853–1859.

Russcher H, Smit P, van Rossum EFC, van den Akker ELT, et al. Strategies for the characterization of disorders in cortisol sensitivity. J Clin Endocrinol Metab. 2006; 91(2):694-701.

Schelling G, Stoll C, Kapfhammer HP, et al. The effect of stress doses of hydrocortisone during septic shock on posttraumatic stress disorder and health-related quality of life in survivors. Crit Care Med. 1999;27:2678–2683.

Schelling G, Briegel J, Roozendaal B, et al. The effect of stress doses of hydrocortisone during septic shock on posttraumatic stress disorder in survivors. Biol Psychiatr. 2001;50:978–985.

LENA D. EDWARDS MD, FAARM

Schuder SE. Stress-induced hypocortisolemia diagnosed as psychiatric disorders responsive to hydrocortisone replacement. Ann NY Acad Sci. 2006;1057:466-478.

Scott LV, Teh J, Reznek R, Martin A, et al. Small adrenal glands in chronic fatigue syndrome: a preliminary computer tomography study. Psychoneuroendocrinology. 1999;24:759-768.

Sephton S, Sapolsky R, Kraemer H, Spiegel D. Diurnal cortisol rhythm as a predictor of breast cancer survival. J Natl Cancer Inst. 2000;92:994–1000.

Sudhaus S, et al. Salivary cortisol and psychological mechanisms in patients with acute versus chronic low back pain. Psychoneuroendocrinology. 2009 May;34(4):513-22.

Simunkova K, Hampl R, Hill M, Kriz L, Hrda P, et al. Adrenocortical function in young adults with diabetes mellitus type 1. J Steroid Biochem Mol Biol. 2010 Oct;122(1-3):35-41.

Sternberg J. Neuroendocrine regulation of autoimmune/inflammatory disease. Endocrinol. 2001;169:429–435,.

Terzidis K, Panoutsopoulos A, Mantzou A, Tourli P, Papageorgiou G, et al. Lower early morning plasma cortisol levels are associated with thyroid autoimmunity in the elderly. Eur J Endocrinol. 2010;162:307-313.

Tops M, Riese H, Oldehinkel AJ, Rijsdijk FV, Ormel J. Rejection sensitivity relates to hypocortisolism and depressed mood state in young women. Psychoneuroendocrinology. 2008;33:551-559.

Van Hoof E, Cluydts R, De Meirleir K. Atypical depression as a secondary symptom in chronic fatigue syndrome. Med. Hypotheses. 2003;61:52-55.

Van Houdenhove B, Egle U, Luyten P. The role of life stress in fibromyalgia. Curr Rheumatol Rep. 2005 Oct;7(5):365-70.

Wirtz PH, von Kanel R, Emini L, Ruedisueli K, Groessbauer S, et al. Evidence for altered hypothalamus-pituitary-adrenal axis functioning in systemic hypertension: Blunted cortisol response to awakening and lower negative feedback sensitivity. Psychoneuroendocrinology. 2007;32:430-436.

Wolfe F, Smythe HA, Yunus MB, Bennett RM, Bombardier C, et al. The American College of Rheumatology 1990 Criteria for the Classification of Fibromyalgia. Report of the Multicenter Criteria Committee. Arthritis Rheum. 1990;33:160–72.

Wolfe F. Fibromyalgia: The clinical syndrome. Rheum Dis Clin North Am. 1989;15:1–18.

Yehuda R. Sensitization of the hypothalamic-pituitary-adrenal axis in posttraumatic stress disorder. Ann NY Acad Sci. 1997;821:57-75.

World Health Organization Fact Sheet: http://www.who.int/nmh/publications/fact_sheet_cancers_en.pdf

CHAPTER NINE

Anton PA. Stress and mind-body impact on the course of inflammatory bowel diseases. Semin Gastrointest Dis. 1999 Jan;10(1):14-9.

Bafna PA, Balaraman R. Anti-ulcer and anti-oxidant activity of pepticare, a herbomineral formulation. Phytomedicine. 2005;2(4):264-70.

Baran SE, Campbell AM, Kleen JK, Foltz CH, Wright RL, Diamond DM, Conrad CD. Combination of high fat diet and chronic stress retracts hippocampal dendrites. Neuroreport. 2005 Jan 19;16(1):39-43.

Berdyshev V, Breckmann II (ed). Int Collection of Scientific Papers, Issue 2, Vladivostok, Dalnauka, 105-117.

Berdyshev VV. Some specific effects of single doses of adaptogens. In Valeology: Diagnois, Means and Practice in Healthcare, Breckmann II (ed). Int Collection of Scientific Papers, Issue 2, Vladivostok, Dalnauka, 105-117.

Bleakney TL. Deconstructing an adaptogen: Eleutherococcus senticosus. Holist Nurs Pract. 2008 Jul-Aug;22(4):220-4.

Blumenthal M. The ABC Clinical Guide to Herbs. Austin, TX. American Botanical Council; 2003:97–106.

Brown RP, Gerbarg PL. Yoga breathing, meditation, and longevity. Ann N Y Acad Sci. 2009 Aug;1172:54-62.

Choi Kwang-tae. Botanical characteristics, pharmacological effects and medicinal components of Korean Panax Ginseng C A Meyer. Acta Pharmacol Sin. 2008;29(9): 1009-1118.

Chiou WF, Chang PC, et al., Protein constituent contributes to the hypotensive and vasrelaxant activities of Cordyceps sinensis. Life Sci. 2000 Feb 25;66(14):1369-1376.

Cleare AJ, Heap E, Malhi GS, Wessely S, O'Keane V, Miell J. Low dose hydrocortisone in chronic fatigue syndrome: a randomized crossover trial. The Lancet. 1999;353:455-458.

Clifford, T. 1990. Tibetan Buddhist Medicine and Psychiatry: 84. Samuel Weiser, Inc. York Beach, ME.

Dasgupta T, Rao AR, Yadava PK. Chemomodulatory efficacy of basil leaf (Ocimum basilicum) on drug metabolizing and antioxidant enzymes, and on carcinogen-induced skin and forestomach papillomagenesis. Phytomedicine. 2004 Feb; 11(2-3):139-51.

Davydov M, Krikorian AD. Eleutherococcus senticosus (Rupr. & Maxim.) Maxim. Araliaceae) as an adaptogen: a closer look. J Ethnopharmacol. 2000;72:345-393.

De Bock K, Eijnde BO, et al. Acute Rhodiola rosea intake can improve endurance exercise performance. Int J Sport Nutr Exerc Metab. 2004;14:298-307.

Demitrack MA, Engleberg NC. Chronic fatigue syndrome. Curr Ther Endocrinol Metab. 1994;5:135-142.

Dhingra D, Parle M, and Kulkarni SK, Memory enhancing activity of Glycyrrhiza glabra in mice. J Ethnopharmacol. 2004;91:361-5.

Fahey TD, Pearl MD. The hormonal and perceptive effects of phosphatidylersine administration during two weeks of resistive exercise-induced overtraining. Biol Sport. 1998;15:135-144.

Feuerstein, G. 1998. The yoga tradition: its history, literature, philosophy, and practice. Hohm Press. Prescott, AZ.

Fukuda K, Straus S, Hickie I. The chronic fatigue syndrome: a comprehensive approach to its treatment and study. Ann Int Med. 1994;12:953-959.

Goldbart AD, Row BW, Kheirandish-Gozal L, Cheng Y, Brittian KR, Gozal D. High fat/refined carbohydrate diet enhances the susceptibility to spatial learning deficits in rats exposed to intermittent hypoxia. Brain Res. 2006;1090 (1):190-6.

Golf SW, Bender S, Grüttner J. On the significance of magnesium in extreme physical stress. Cardiovascular Drugs and Therapy. 1998;12:197-202.

Hannan JM, Marenah L, et al. Ocimum sanctum leaf extracts stimulate insulin secretion from perfused pancreas, isolated islets and clonal pancreatic beta-cells. J Endocrinol. 2006;189(1):127-36.

Haraguchi H, Yoshida N, et al. Protection of mitochondrial functions against oxidative stresses by isoflavans from Glycyrrhiza glabra. J Pharm Pharmacol 2000;52(2):219-23.

Head KA, Kelly GS. Nutrients and botanicals for treatment of stress: adrenal fatigue, neurotransmitter imbalance, anxiety, and restless sleep. Altern Med Rev. 2009 Jun; 14 (2):114-40.

Holtorf KH. Diagnosis and treatment of hypothalamic-pituitary-adrenal (hpa) axis dysfunction in patients with chronic fatigue syndrome (CFS) and fibromyalgia (FM) J Chronic Fatigue Syn. 2008;14(3):1-14.

Infante JR, Peran F, Martinez M, Roldan A, Poyatos R, Ruiz C, Samaniego F, Garrido F. ACTH and beta-endorphin in transcendental meditation. Physiol Behav. 1998 Jun 1;64(3):311-5.

The International Agency for Research on Cancer (IARC). http://monographs.iarc.fr/ENG/Monographs/vol98/mono98-8E.pdf

Jayasinghe C, Gotoh N, Aoki T, Wada S. Phenolics composition and antioxidant activity of sweet basil (osimum basilicum). J Agric Food Chem. 2003 July 16;51 (15):4442-9.

Kakude T. Neuroprotective effects of the green tea components theanine and catechins. Biol Pharm Bull. 2002;25:1513-1518.

Kalman DS, Feldman S, et al. Effect of a proprietary Magnolia and Phellodendron extract on stress levels in healthy women: a pilot, double-blind, placebo-controlled clinical trial. Nutr J. 2008 Apr 21;7:11.

Kanoski SE, Meisel RL, Mullins AJ, Davidson TL. The effects of energy-rich diets on discrimination reversal learning and on BDNF in the hippocampus and prefrontal cortex of the rat. Behav Brain Res. 2007 Aug 22;182(1):57-66.

Kelly GS. Nutritional and botanical interventions to assist with the adaptation to stress. Altern Med Rev. 1999 Aug;4(4):249-65.

Komar VV, Kit SM, Sishchuk LV. Effect of Rhodiola rosea on human mental activity. Pharm J. 1981;36:62-62.

Kucinskaite A, Briedis V, Savickas A, Experimental analysis of therapeutic properties of Rhodiola rosea L. and its possible application in medicine. Medicina (Kaunas). 2004 Jan; 40:614-619.

Lee YJ, Lee YM, Lee CK, Jung JK, Han SB, Hong JT. Therapeutic applications of compounds in the Magnolia family. Pharmacol Ther. 2011 May;130(2):157-76.

Mattioli L, Perfumi M. Rhodiola rosea L. extract reduces stress- and CRF-induced anorexia in rats. J Psychopharmacol. 2007 Sep;21(7):742-50.

McCarthy MF. Prenatal high-dose pyridoxine may prevent hypertension and syndrome X in-utero by protecting the fetus from excess glucocorticoid activity. Med Hypotheses. 2000 May;54(5):808-13.

Mishra LC, Singh BB, Dagenais S. Scientific basis for the therapeutic use of Withania somnifera (ashwagandha): a review. Altern Med Rev. 2000;(4):334-46.

Mohanty I, Arya DS, et al, Mechanisms of cardioprotective effect of Withania somnifera in experimentally induced myocardial infarction. 2004;94(4):184-90.

Murck H; Steiger A. Mg2+ reduces ACTH secretion and enhances spindle power without changing delta power during sleep in men - possible therapeutic implications. Psychopharmacology. 1998;137(3):247-52.

National Center for Health Statistics: "NCHS Data Brief No. 42, September 2010." Olsson EMG, von Scheele B, Panossian AG. A randomized, double-blind, placebo-controlled, parallel-group study of the standardized extract of SHR-5 of the roots of Rhodiola rosea in the treatment of subjects with stress-related fatigue. Plant Med. 2009;75:105-112.

Onuki M, Suzawa A. Effect of pantethine on the function of the adrenal cortex. 2. Clinical experience using pantethine in cases under steroid hormone treatment. Horumon To Rinsho. 1970;18:937-940.

LENA D. EDWARDS MD, FAARM

Pace TW, Negi LT, Adame DD, Cole SP, Sivilli TI, Brown TD, Issa MJ, Raison CL. Effect of compassion meditation on neuroendocrine, innate immune and behavioral responses to psychosocial stress. Psychoneuroendocrinology. 2009;34:87-98.

Panossian A, Wagner H. Stimulating effect of adaptogens: an overview with particular reference to their efficacy following single dose administration. Phytother Res. 2005; 19:819-838.

Panossian A, Wikman G. Evidence-based efficacy of adaptogens in fatigue, and molecular mechanisms related to their stress-protective activity. Curr Clin Pharmacol. 2009 Sep;4(3):198-219.

Panossian A, Wikman G. Pharmacology of Schisandra chinensis Bail: an overview of Russian research and uses in medicine. J Ethnopharmacol. 2008 Jul 23;118(2):183-212.

Panossian et al. Plant adaptogens. III. Earlier and more recent aspects and concepts on their mode of action. Phytomedicine. 1999;6:147-155.

Panossian et al. Stimulating effect of adaptogens: an overview with particular reference to their efficacy following single dose administration. Phytother Res. 2005; 19:819-838.

Park SK, Jung IC, Lee WK, Lee YS, Park HK, Go HJ, Kim K, Lim NK, Hong JT, Ly SY, Rho SS. A combination of green tea extract and l-theanine improves memory and attention in subjects with mild cognitive impairment: a double-blind placebo-controlled study. J Med Food. 2011 Apr;14(4):334-43.

Rayssiguier Y, Libako P, Nowacki W, Rock E. Magnesium deficiency and metabolic syndrome: stress and inflammation may reflect calcium activation. Magnes Res. 2010 Jun;23(2):73-80.

Sarris J. Herbal medicines in the treatment of psychiatric disorders: a systematic review. Phytother Res. 2007 Aug;21(8):703-16.

Straub RH, Schölmerich J, Zietz B. Replacement therapy with DHEA plus corticosteroids in patients with chronic inflammatory diseases--substitutes of adrenal and sex hormones. J Rheumatol. 2000; 59 Suppl 2:II/108-18.

Shelygina NM et al. Influence of Vitamins C, Bl, and B6 on the diurnal periodicity of the glucocorticoid function of the adrenal cortex in patients with atherosclerotic cardiosclerosis. AbstractVopr Pitan. 1975 Mar-Apr;(2):25-9.

Streeter CC, Whitfield TH, Owen L, Rein T et al. Effects of yoga versus walking on mood, anxiety, and brain GABA levels: a randomized controlled MRS study. J Altern Complement Med. 2010 Nov;16(11):1145-52.

Theise ND. Beyond cell doctrine: complexity theory informs alternate models of the body for cross-cultural dialogue. Ann N Y Acad Sci. 2009 Aug;1172:263-9.

Vinogradov VV, Tarasov IuA, Tishin VS, Bogdanovich VI, Spas VV.[Thiamine prevention of the corticosteroid reaction afer surgery]. Probl Endokrinol (Mosk). 1981 May-Jun;27(3):11-6.

Walton KG et al. Lowering cortisol and CVD risk in postmenopausal women: a pilot study using the Transcendental Meditation program. Ann NY Acad Sci. 2004;1032:211-5.

Winston & Maimes. Adaptogens: Herbs for Strength, Stamina, and Stress Relief. Healing Arts Press. 2007.

Winters M. Ancient medicine, modern use: Withania somnifera and its potential role in integrative oncology. Alt Med Review. 2006;11(4):269-77.

Zhu JS, Halpern GM, Jones K. The scientific rediscovery of a precious ancient Chinese herbal regimen: Cordyceps sinensis: part II. J Altern Complement Med. 1998 Dec 1;4(4):429-457.

LENA D. EDWARDS MD. FAARM

GLOSSARY

ACTH (adrenocorticotropic hormone)
The pituitary hormone responsible for directly affecting the regulation and release of cortisol and other adrenal gland hormones.

ADAPTIVE/ADAPTATION
An internal change which occurs under the influence of external changes in order to maintain the function of tissues and organ systems. Although adaptation allows for survival, optimal physiological processes and functions are often compromised.

ADENOPATHY
The medical term for enlarged and inflamed lymph nodes.

ADRENAL CORTICOSTEROID PRODUCTION
Corticosteroid (hormone) produced by the adrenal glands.

ANTIOCICEPTIVE
A term used to describe a substance that reduces one's sensitivity to pain.

ANTI-NEOPLASTIC
A term used to describe anything that helps in preventing the formation of cells capable of becoming cancerous.

ANTI-OXIDANT
A molecule whose function is to prevent 'oxidation' (equivalent to the process of 'rusting' on the inside of your body). Cells are damaged during the process of oxidation which can ultimately lead to DNA damage (cancer and other diseases) or cell death. Vitamins E and C, glutathione, and lipoic acid are some examples of anti-oxidants.

CATECHOLAMINES
The collective name given to hormones of the sympathetic nervous system

(SNS) which include epinephrine and norepinephrine They are released by the adrenal glands when the SNS is activated by a stressor.

CIRCADIAN RHYTHMS
An individual's natural internal sleep/wake-related rhythms which occur throughout a 24-hour period.

DHEA (dehydroepiandrosterone)
An important adrenal gland hormone involved in many aspects of optimal bodily function and disease prevention. Not only does it keep the activity of cortisol in check (cortisol antagonist), it also serves as a very important pro-hormone in the production of the sex hormones (estrogen, progesterone, testosterone), particularly in postmenopausal women.

DOPAMINE
An important neurotransmitter produced in the brain from the amino acid tyrosine. Although it has many important functions in its own right, it is also the precursor to the production of catecholamines and has an inhibitory affect on cortisol production and function.

EPIDEMIOLOGICAL
The study of patterns of health, illness, and associated factors within populations.

EPINEPHRINE (also known as adrenalin)
One of the two primary hormones in the catecholamines family. Epinephrine, which is made from the neurotransmitter Dopamine, is produced only by the adrenal glands. It is rapidly released during stressful events, particularly physical stress, noise, and temperature changes. This hormone prepares the body for its "fight or flight" response by causing an increase in blood pressure and heart rate and causes an increase in blood sugar by increasing liver glucose production and amino acid breakdown in the muscles.

FSH (folliculefollicle stimulating hormone)
A hormone produced by the pituitary gland which is responsible for stimulation of egg formation and production of estrogen in women. In

men, its function is to stimulate the production of sperm.

FUNCTIONAL HYPOTHYROIDISM
Also known as 'subclinical hypothyroidism' or 'euthyroid sick syndrome', functional hypothyroidism represents the presence of signs and symptoms of low thyroid in the absence of abnormal test results.

HIPPOCAMPUS
A horseshoe shaped expanse of neurons located in the temporal lobes of the brain. It serves an essential role in formation and retention of memories, spatial orientation, navigation, and emotions.

HYPOTHALAMUS
The primary central regulator of hormone production. It is responsible for producing various 'releasing hormones' which then tell other glands and tissues to produce stimulating hormones.

HYPOTHALAMIC-PITUITARY-ADRENAL (HPA) axis
The term used to describe the complex interactions and effects of the major components of the stress response system, namely the hypothalamus, the pituitary gland, and the adrenal glands. Under other hormonal and bodily influences, this axis ultimately determines the body's response to stress.

IDIOPATHIC
A condition without an identifiable cause or source.

IMMUNE SYSTEM
An under appreciated but extremely influential component of the stress response system. Not only does the immune system directly affect the release of stress hormones, cortisol and DHEA in particular, but the function and activity of the immune system is directly affected by the presence or absence of these hormones as well.

INOSITOL
A natural compound found in the body (and also found in food such as fruits and nuts). Supplementation with inositol may be helpful in reducing anxiety, depression and promoting sleep.

LENA D. EDWARDS MD, FAARM

LOW DOSE NALTREXONE (LDN)

A medicine traditionally used in higher doses to curb cravings for alcohol. Lower doses have been shown to be beneficial in some autoimmune diseases (multiple sclerosis, Crohn's disease), as well as in infectious diseases and infertility.

LH (luteinizing hormone)

Produced in the pituitary gland, this hormone 'surges' during a woman's cycle to stimulate ovulation. Males benefit from the actions of this hormone on the cells in the testes responsible for testosterone production.

MYALGIA

The medical term for muscle pain.

NEUROPROTECTIVE

A term used to describe anything that supports brain function and protects it from damage and disease.

NEUROTRANSMITTERS

Chemicals released from nerve cells that serve as a communication medium within the nervous system. The neurologic messages carried by these chemicals are relayed from the nerve cells to other tissues of the body.

NOREPINEPHRINE

The second major catecholamine, it is produced in several areas throughout the body including the adrenal glands. It works in conjunction with epinephrine to initiate the immediate "fight or flight" response. Its primary effects are to mobilize glucose from energy stores, to directly increase heart rate, and to increase blood flow to muscles.

OXIDATIVE STRESS

The term used to describe the body's inability to overcome its natural ability to neutralize the constant, low levels of oxidation (akin to the process of rusting) which occurs as a result of the accumulation of 'free radicals' (activated oxygen molecules that are harmful to tissues). Over time, oxidative stress can result in cell and tissue damage and even death which culminates in the form of premature aging, diseases, and possibly premature death.

PATHOPHYSIOLOGY
The study of the physical signs and symptoms of a disease as it relates to the underlying abnormalities at the cell and tissue levels.

PHARMACEUTICAL GRADE
The classification assigned a supplement that has been found to follow certain guidelines to ensure the content, purity, potency, and safety. Pharmaceutical grade supplements are 99 percent pure without additives or unnecessary substances which may cause unwanted side effects.

PHYSIOLOGICAL
Consistent with the normal and optimal function of cells, tissues, and organs.

PITUITARY GLAND
Produces ACTH (adrenocorticotropic hormone) which then commands the adrenal glands to produce the stress hormones. The pituitary gland is also responsible for producing growth hormone, stimulating hormones which control the release of thyroid hormones and reproductive hormones, and other hormones.

PMS (premenstrual syndrome)
The constellation of emotional and physical symptoms which occurs in females one to two weeks prior to the onset of menstruation.

PREGNENOLONE
A hormone at the top of the steroid hormone production chain which serves as precursor to all steroid hormones, including cortisol and DHEA. It is produced mainly in the adrenals and the brain. It also serves as an anti-inflammatory hormone, preserves memory, and positively influences electrical communication in the brain.

PROBIOTIC
Beneficial bacteria and/or yeast which restore optimal populations of healthy organisms within the intestinal tract thereby aiding food digestion, improving nutritional absorption, and reducing 'gut' inflammation.

LENA D. EDWARDS MD. FAARM

PROGESTINS

A group of synthetically produced hormones with actions similar to progesterone. However, structurally and functionally, progestins are not identical to our body's own progesterone. Consequently, they may cause detrimental side effects such as breast cancer. They have been traditionally used as a component of oral contraceptives since, unlike natural progesterone, progestins suppress ovulation.

RECEPTOR

A protein on the surface of a cell to which a hormone must bind in order for its effects to be either turned on or turned off. Many hormones can 'cross bind' to other hormone receptors (for instance, cortisol can also bind to aldosterone receptors). Often, tissues have multiple different sub-types of receptors for one hormone. This is important because the same hormone can cause different effects in different tissues depending upon the sub-type and number of receptors present.

SALIVARY CORTISOL PATTERNS

The pattern of cortisol release as demonstrated through analysis of saliva. This is often done at four specific points throughout the day.

SOMATOFORM

A mental disorder characterized by complaints of physical illness without any identifiable physical or laboratory abnormality to corroborate the physical complaints.

RECOMMENDED RESOURCES

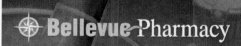
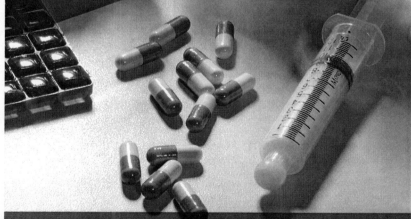

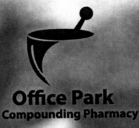

RECOMMENDED RESOURCES

- The American Institute of Stress
- National Institute of Occupational Safety and Health (NIOSH)
- International Stress Management Association (ISMA)
- American Psychological Association (APA)
- World Health Organization (WHO)
- The Institute for Stress Management and Performance Improvement
- Canadian Institute of Stress
- The Stress Management Society (UK)
- American Academy of Anti-Aging Medicine (A4M)
- National Institutes of Health
- American College for Advancement in Medicine
- The Center for Mind Body Medicine
- National Center for Complementary and Alternative Medicine